"*The Mind-Gut Connection* presents the incredibly humbling reality that our very perception and interpretation of the world around us is virtually dictated by the microbes living within us. This book redefines what it means to be healthy and eloquently provides the means to manifest that goal."
—David Perlmutter, MD, author of the #1 *New York Times* bestseller *Grain Brain* and *Brain Maker*

"Drawing on his vast experience as a practicing gastroenterologist, Dr. Mayer writes about the connections that our brains have with our guts, especially with the microbes that make the gut their home. Describing a rapidly advancing realm of knowledge, this thoughtful guide provides practical advice to improve health."
—Martin J. Blaser, MD, author of *Missing Microbes*

"Dr. Emeran Mayer elucidates the intricate biochemical dialogue that occurs between the brain, digestive tract, and trillions of bacteria residing in the gut. He dubs this form of communication 'microbe-speak' and speculates on its implications for social behavior, decision-making, emotional well-being, and maybe mental health."   —*Booklist*

"After a long period of neglect the enteric nervous system has been recognized as the 'second brain'. Dr. Emeran Mayer, a true expert of this topic, has now written the best lay-public guide yet to this spectacular part of ourselves. Recommended reading."   —Antonio Demasio, author of *Descartes' Error, The Feeling of What Happens,* and *The Self Comes to Mind*

"I have known Emeran Mayer for years and have learned to pay attention to what he says and writes. *The Mind-Gut Connection* is a delight. Both scholarly and fun to read, I highly recommend it to anyone interested in learning more about how the mind and gut communicate."

—Michael D. Gershon, MD, author of *The Second Brain*

"Microbiome research is revolutionizing our understanding of the human body and the brain. In *The Mind-Gut Connection*, Dr. Emeran Mayer provides authoritative insight into this rapidly expanding field. Synthesizing recent research with patient stories and personal anecdotes, he offers practical, evidence-based recommendations to keep the dialogue between the brain, the gut, and its microbes flowing smoothly."

—Rob Knight, PhD, author of *Follow Your Gut*
and director of the Center for Microbiome Innovation,
University of California San Diego

"*The Mind-Gut Connection* is a revolutionary new holistic view of what keeps us healthy, ranging from the food choices we make to the ways we can train our mind, with the ultimate goal of attaining optimal health."

—Kenneth R. Pelletier, PhD, MD, Clinical Professor of
Medicine and Professor of Public Health,
University of California School of Medicine (UCSF)

"We are perennially drawn to research on the gut but Dr. Mayer is really writing for anyone looking to understand how their body works, and (most importantly) how to retrain their two brains to communicate better." —*Goop*

THE
Mind-Gut
CONNECTION

THE
Mind-Gut
CONNECTION

How the Hidden Conversation
Within Our Bodies Impacts Our Mood,
Our Choices, and Our Overall Health

Dr. Emeran Mayer

HARPER WAVE

An Imprint of HarperCollins*Publishers*

FIRST HARPER WAVE PAPERBACK EDITION PUBLISHED 2018.

Designed by Leah Carlson-Stanisic

Illustration by © Barmaleeva/Getty Images

Library of Congress Cataloging-in-Publication Data has been applied for.

ISBN 978-0-06-237658-9 (pbk.)

23 24 25 26 27 LBC 41 40 39 38 37

To Minou and Dylan
for their persistent encouragement to
listen to my gut feelings.

To my mentor, John H. Walsh,
who kindled my interest in gut-brain communications.

CONTENTS

IIIIIIIIIIIIIIIIIIIIIIIIIIIIIIIIIIIIIIII

Part 1
OUR BODY, THE INTELLIGENT SUPERCOMPUTER

Part 2
INTUITION AND GUT FEELINGS

Part 3
HOW TO OPTIMIZE BRAIN–GUT HEALTH

PREFACE

||||||||||||||||||||||||||||||||||||||||||||||||||||||||||||||||||||||||||||||||||||||||||||||||||||||||||||||||||||||||||||||||

Since the initial publication of *The Mind-Gut Connection* in the summer of 2016, I have talked to many audiences large and small, to the lay public and to academics across America and Europe, on the topic of brain-gut interactions and how our gut health impacts our overall mental and physical health. I've also met one-on-one with many readers interested in learning more about how this emerging science can improve their overall well-being and, for some, their daily quality of life.

Many of these individuals were patients who recognized their own or their child's symptoms in the stories I share in the book. Some were seeking advice on how best to harness the recent insights into the microbiome to alleviate digestive symptoms, improve their anxiety or depression, or slow the progression of neurological diseases such as Parkinson's. Others were executives from the burgeoning biotech industry or the food industry looking for guidance on how to tailor their products to promote microbiome health.

These experiences have convinced me that the so-called "brain-gut-microbiome axis" and its impact on our mood and our health has become a hot topic. Every day more and more scientific literature offers evidence that disturbances of brain-gut interaction have implications for a wide array of health issues, from conditions like food sensitivities and functional GI disorders to psychiatric disorders like depression and food addiction to brain disorders like autism spectrum disorders, Alzheimer's disease, and Parkinson's disease. While some of these ideas and hypotheses about specific brain disorders remain speculative, a few are now supported by well-designed studies in human subjects.

For example, in the short amount of time since the *The Mind-Gut Connection* was published, four studies have been published that have clearly linked an alteration in gut microbial composition in patients with chronic depression. However, it is important to keep in mind that the majority of published human studies so far have only demonstrated *associations* between alterations in gut microbial composition and specific diagnoses, without proving a causal relationship. In other words, we don't know if the observed changes in the gut microbiome in these diseases are a cause of the respective disease or a consequence of the underlying brain disorder, altered disease-related dietary patterns, or medication use. But it's clear that there is a connection between the microbiome and cognitive function. Well-designed research is now underway to determine possible causality and to identify novel targets for the treatment of common brain disorders.

Of the various aspects of the brain-gut microbiome communication addressed in *The Mind-Gut Connection*, I receive the most feedback and questions on the topic of nutrition. It wasn't until I started having conversations with readers that I realized how challenging it has become for health-minded people to determine which foods are right for them. Given the array of food information and diets available—many with contradictory messages—how can one decide what eating style is best? There is an ever-growing number of books and websites promoting these conflicting messages supposedly based on the latest scientific evidence, and often these messages are linked to online shopping sites for food supplements, including pre- and probiotics. How should a health-conscious person decide if it is better to consume a mix of ten ("carefully selected") different probiotic strains (as recommended on various websites) and if it is important to buy a probiotic with more than 40 billion CFU (colony-forming units)? Despite the information provided online, including Amazon reviews (the majority of which are paid advertisements), surprisingly there is currently no scientific evidence to prove the great majority of these claims. If the confused patient turns to his or her doctor for advice, he or she will likely be disappointed. The majority of healthcare providers are neither on top of the rapidly progressing science of the microbiome, nor trained in giving evidence-based nutritional advice.

By focusing on the detrimental effects of the modern North American diet in *The Mind-Gut Connection*, it became obvious to me that a diet that is high in plant-based complex carbohydrates (from a large variety of different plants), plant-derived fat, grains, naturally fermented foods, and fish, and low in red meat, animal-derived fat, refined sugars, and processed food is the blueprint for most healthy diets around the world. Even better, if you add the benefits of polyphenols (molecules with health-promoting effects that are largely processed by the gut microbiota) contained in olive oil and red wine, certain plant products with anti-inflammatory effects such as turmeric, curcumin, and ginger, and a large number of fermented foods teeming with microorganisms, you have a simple road map for a diet that is good for your microbes (increases the diversity, abundance, and populations of health-promoting microbes), good for your gut (reduces intestinal permeability, e.g., improves a leaky gut), and good for your brain (prevents low-grade immune activation in your brain). While as a scientist, I rarely give up my professional skepticism toward new health benefit claims of any treatment, in the case of dietary and lifestyle recommendations based on the new brain-gut microbiome science, I am willing to drop my skepticism and unconditionally endorse such a way of eating.

In *The Mind-Gut Connection*, I focused on the Mediterranean diet as an example of an eating style with significant evidence-based health benefit for us and our gut microbes. Based on this growing scientific evidence, studies are now underway evaluating the benefits of the Mediterranean diet for slowing the progression of Alzheimer's and Parkinson's disease, or for the improved pharmacologic treatment of depression. Such studies would have been unthinkable and unfundable even ten years ago, before the science of the microbiome became available.

While I have focused on the example of the Mediterranean diet in this book, it is certainly not the only diet that is associated with gut and brain health benefits. Most traditional diets all around the world share a similar composition to the Mediterranean diet, even though the individual ingredients may vary depending on the respective geographic region. Traditional Asian diets, for example, including the Japanese, Korean, and Chinese diets, share a high consumption of fish, varied plant-based foods rich in polyphenols and antioxidants, grains, and naturally fermented foods, and limited meat and dairy products. In addition, traditional food consumption in these Asian cultures as well as in Mediterranean countries has a strong communal element, including the sharing of multiple small dishes during a meal.

During a trip to Korea in the fall of 2016, I learned that the traditional Korean diet consisted, to a large degree, of plant-based dishes, fish, and poultry with a moderate amount of red meat and very little animal-based fat. And then there was the eye-opening experience of seeing the numerous fermented foods that accompanied the main dish; for every meal, there was an astonishing number and variety of so-called fermented banchan, kimchi, and kimchi soup. After three days of enjoying these traditional Korean dishes, including up to thirty different types of banchan along with rice and soup, I started to wonder how many live microorganisms the average Koreans must ingest every year starting from infancy, a period that is particularly critical for the formation of a healthy microbiome and the brain-gut axis.

In Japan, a traditional meal may consist of a bowl of miso soup, a bowl of rice, some fish, and several vegetable dishes—cooked, fried, or pickled—all served on small plates. This way of eating and often sharing multiple, small portions resembles the way Koreans eat their fermented banchan and people in Spain enjoy their tapas. Another important element of the Japanese cuisine is the mindfulness that goes both into the artful preparation of the meal and its consumption. Traditional food in Japan is not something that is consumed while driving in the car or watching TV, and it is not valued based on its quantity or macronutrient composition. As I experienced during my visits to Japan, eating a Japanese meal fully engages one's attention, appealing to all the senses, including visual appeal, texture, and taste.

The benefits for longevity, cardiovascular health, and brain health of the traditional Japanese diet are well established. An increase in the prevalence of typical Western diseases such as obesity, metabolic syndrome, and Alzheimer's disease have significantly increased in Japanese living in the United States, approximating rates seen in non-Japanese Americans. But also for Japanese not living in the United States, the prevalence of dementia has increased over the last few decades. Proposed mechanisms to explain this phenomenon in Japan include the gradual shift away from fish and mainly plant-based foods to a higher consumption of meat and animal products. Data suggests that one dietary factor most strongly associated with the rise in Alzheimer's disease in Japan is the increased consumption of animal fat.

There are other populations around the world which illustrate the negative impact on people's health when shifting from a largely plant-based diet to the North American diet. Well-documented population studies on dietary habits and chronic disease exist to show the detrimental effect of these dietary shifts on the metabolic and brain health of Hawaiians, Native Americans, and indigenous populations in Central America.

It is intriguing to speculate, even though not proven at this point, that the health benefits of the Japanese diet and other traditional diets around the world have something to do with their positive influence on the composition and diversity of the gut microbiota. As I discuss extensively in this book, plant-based diets are associated with a healthier gut microbiome, and with a greatly reduced risk for low-grade inflammation throughout the body, including the brain. I strongly believe that the health benefits of the traditional Japanese diet, including the Okinawan diet, are to a significant degree a consequence of an optimal regulation of the interactions between diet, the gut microbiome, and the gut.

I hope that the reader will find this book helpful not only in gaining a better understanding of the ways in which the brain, gut, and microbiome communicate with each other in health and disease but also in making more rational and science-based decisions about what to eat to stay well. While it will take a long time before we fully understand the complexities of the gut microbiome and its interactions with our brain, the simple recommendations in this book can be implemented immediately.

Emeran A. Mayer
Los Angeles, California
August 14, 2017

THE
Mind-Gut
CONNECTION

PART 1

||||||||||||||||||||||||||||||||

OUR BODY, THE
INTELLIGENT
SUPERCOMPUTER

CHAPTER

1

THE MIND-BODY
CONNECTION IS REAL

||||||||||||||||||||||||||||||||||||||||||||||||||||||||||||||||||||||||||||||||||||||||||||||||||||||||||||||||||||||||||||||||

When I started medical school in 1970, doctors looked at the human body as a complicated machine with a finite number of independent parts. On average, it functioned for about seventy-five years, provided you took care of it and fed it the right fuel. Like a high-quality car, it ran well, provided that it didn't have any major accidents, and that no parts were irreversibly compromised or broken. A few routine checkups during a lifetime were all you were expected to do to prevent any unexpected calamities. Medicine and surgery provided powerful tools to fix acute problems, such as infections, accidental injuries, or heart disease.

However, over the past forty to fifty years, something fundamental has gone wrong with our health, and the old model no longer seems to be able to provide an explanation or a solution of how to fix the problems. What's happening can no longer be easily explained simply by a single malfunctioning organ or gene. Instead, we are beginning to realize that the complex regulatory mechanisms that help our bodies and brains adapt to our rapidly changing environment are in turn being impacted by our changing lifestyles. These mechanisms do not operate independently, but as parts of a whole. They regulate our food intake, metabolism and body weight, our immune system, and the development and health of our brains. We are just beginning to realize that the gut, the microbes living in it—the gut microbiota—and the signaling molecules that they produce from their vast number of genes—the microbiome—constitute one of the major components of these regulatory systems.

In this book, I will offer a revolutionary new look at how the brain, the gut, and the trillions of microorganisms living in the gut communicate with each other. In particular, I will focus on the role these connections play in maintaining the health of our brain and our gut. I will discuss the negative consequences on the health of these two organs when their cross talk is disturbed, and propose ways of how to obtain optimal health by reestablishing and optimizing brain-gut communications.

Even in medical school, the traditional, prevailing approach did not sit quite right with me. Despite all the studying of organ systems and disease mechanisms, I was surprised that there rarely was any mention of the brain and its possible involvement in such common diseases as stomach ulcers, hypertension, or chronic pain. In addition, I had seen a number of patients during rounds in the hospital for whom even the most thorough diagnostic investigations failed to reveal a cause of their symptoms. These symptoms mostly had to do with chronic pain experienced in different areas of the body: in the belly, the pelvic area, and the chest. So, in my third year of medical school, when it was time to begin my dissertation, I wanted to study the biology of how the brain interacted with the body, in the hope that I would develop a better understanding of many of these common diseases. Over a period of several months, I approached several professors from different specialties. "Mr. Mayer," said Professor Karl, a senior internal medicine professor at my university, "we all know that the psyche plays an important role in chronic disease. But there is no scientific way today that we can study this clinical phenomenon, and there is certainly no way that you can write a whole dissertation on it."

Professor Karl's disease model, and that of the entire medical system, worked extremely well for certain acute diseases—diseases that come on suddenly, don't last long, or both—in infections, heart attacks, or surgical emergencies like an inflamed appendix. Based on these successes, modern medicine had grown confident. There was hardly an infectious disease left that couldn't be cured by ever-more-powerful antibiotics. Newly developed surgical techniques could prevent and cure many diseases. Broken parts could be removed or replaced. We only needed to figure out all the minute engineering details that made the individual parts of this machine function. Depending more and more on newly evolving technologies, our health care system promoted a pervasive optimism that even the most deadly of chronic health problems, including the scourge of cancer, could be solved eventually.

When President Richard Nixon signed into law the National Cancer Act of 1971, Western medicine acquired a new dimension and a new military metaphor. Cancer became a national enemy, and the human body became a battleground. On that battleground, physicians took a scorched-earth approach to rid the body of disease, using toxic chemicals, deadly radiation, and surgical interventions to attack cancer cells with increasing force. Medicine was already using a similar strategy successfully to combat infectious diseases, unleashing broad-spectrum antibiotics—antibiotics that can kill or cripple many species of bacteria—to wipe out disease-causing bacteria. In both cases, as long as victory could be achieved, collateral damage became an acceptable risk.

For decades, the mechanistic, militaristic disease model set the agenda for medical research: As long as you could fix the affected machine part, we thought, the problem would be solved; there was no need to understand its ultimate cause. This philosophy led to high-blood-pressure treatments that use beta blockers and calcium antagonists to block aberrant signals from the brain to the heart and blood vessels, and proton pump inhibitors that treat gastric ulcers and heartburn by suppressing the stomach's excessive acid production. Medicine and science never paid much attention to the malfunction of the brain that was the primary cause of all these problems. Sometimes the initial approach failed, in which case even more intense efforts were used as a last resort. If the proton pump inhibitor didn't quell the ulcer, you could always cut the entire vagus nerve, the essential bundle of nerve fibers that connects brain and gut.

There is no question that some of these approaches have been remarkably successful, and for years there did not seem to be any need for the medical system and the pharmaceutical industry to change their approach; nor was there much pressure on the patient to prevent the development of the problem in the first place. In particular, there didn't seem to be a need to consider the prominent role of the brain and the distinct signals it sends to the body during stress or negative mind states. The initial remedies for high blood pressure, heart disease, and gastric ulcers were gradually replaced by far more effective treatments that saved lives, reduced suffering, and made the pharmaceutical industry wealthy.

But today, the old mechanistic metaphors are beginning to yield. The machines of forty years ago on which the traditional disease model was based—the cars, ships, and airplanes—had none of the sophisticated computers that play a central role in today's machines. Even the Apollo rockets going to the moon had only rudimentary computing devices on board, millions of times less powerful than an iPhone and more comparable to a Texas Instruments calculator from the 1980s! Not surprisingly, the mechanistic disease models of the day did not include computing power, or intelligence. In other words, they did not consider the brain.

Paralleling the change in technology, the models we use to conceptualize the human body have also changed. Computing power has grown exponentially; cars have become mobile computers on wheels that sense and regulate their parts to ensure proper function, and soon they will drive without human input. Meanwhile, the old fascination with mechanics and engines has given way to a new fascination with information gathering and processing. The machine model was useful in medicine for treating some diseases. But when it comes to understanding chronic diseases of the body and the brain, it's no longer serving us.

The Price Tag of the Machine Model

The traditional view of disease as a breakdown of individual parts of a complex mechanical device that can be fixed by medications or surgery has spawned a continuously growing health care industry. Since 1970, the per capita expense for health care in the United States has increased by more than 2,000 percent. Nearly 20 percent of all goods produced by the U.S. economy per year are required to pay for this enormous undertaking.

But while the World Health Organization, in a landmark report published in 2000, ranked the U.S. health care system as the highest in cost, it ranked it a disappointing 37th in overall performance, and 72nd by overall level of health among 191 member nations included in the study. The United States didn't fare much better in a more recent report by the Commonwealth Fund, which ranked the U.S. health care system as the most expensive per capita among eleven Western countries, about two times higher than all the other surveyed countries. At the same time, the United States came in last in overall performance. This data reflects the hard fact that despite the ever-increasing amount of resources spent on dealing with our nation's health problems, we have made little progress in treating chronic pain conditions, brain-gut disorders such as irritable bowel syndrome (IBS), or mental illnesses such as clinical depression, anxiety, or neurodegenerative disorders. Are we failing because our models for understanding the human body are outdated? There are a growing number of integrative health experts, functional medicine practitioners, and even traditional scientists who would agree with this assumption. But change is on the horizon.

The Mysterious Decline in Our Health

The failure to deal effectively with many chronic diseases, including irritable bowel syndrome, chronic pain, and depression, is not the only shortcoming of the traditional, disease-based model of medicine. Since the 1970s, we have also been witnessing new challenges to our health, including the rapid rise of obesity and related metabolic disorders, autoimmune disorders such as inflammatory bowel diseases, asthma, and allergies, and diseases of the developing and the aging brain, such as autism, Alzheimer's, and Parkinson's disease.

For example, the rate of obesity in the United States has progressively increased from 13 percent of the population in 1972 to 35 percent in 2012. Today 154.7 million American adults are overweight or obese, including 17 percent of American children ages 2 to 19, or 1 in every 6 American children. At least 2.8 million people each year die as a result of being overweight or obese. Globally, 44 percent of diabetes, 23 percent of ischemic heart disease, and 7-41 percent of certain cancers are attributable to overweight and obesity. If the obesity epidemic continues unabated, the costs of treating people suffering from obesity-related diseases are projected to increase to a staggering $620 billion annually

We are still grappling for answers to explain the sudden rise of many of these new health problems, and for most of them, we don't yet have effective solutions. While the increase in our longevity in the United States has paralleled that of many other countries in the developed world, we are far behind in terms of physical and mental well-being when we reach the last decades of our lives. The price we pay for an increase in the quantity of years we live is a decrease in the quality of those years.

In view of these challenges, it's time to update our prevailing model of the human body to understand how it really works, how to keep it running optimally, and how to fix it safely and effectively when something goes wrong. We can no longer tolerate the price tag and the long-term collateral damage that our outdated model has produced.

Until now, we have largely ignored the critical role of two of the most complex and crucial systems in our bodies when it comes to maintaining our overall health: the gut (the digestive system) and the brain (the nervous system). The mind-body connection is far from a myth; it is a biological fact, and an essential link to understand when it comes to our whole body health.

The Supercomputer View of Our Digestive System

For decades, our understanding of the digestive system was based on the machine model of the entire body. It viewed the gut mostly as an old-fashioned device that functioned according to principles of the nineteenth-century steam engine. We ate, chewed and swallowed our food, then our stomach broke it down with mechanical grinding forces assisted by concentrated hydrochloric acid before dumping the homogenized food paste into the small intestine, which absorbed calories and nutrients and sent the undigested food into the large intestine, which disposed of what remained by excreting it. This industrial-age metaphor was easy to grasp, and it influenced generations of doctors, including today's gastroenterologists and surgeons. According to this view, the digestive tract's malfunctioning parts can easily be bypassed or removed, and it can be dramatically rewired to promote weight loss. We have become so skilled in doing these interventions that they can even be performed through an endoscope without surgery.

But as it turns out, this model is overly simplistic. While medicine continues to view the digestive system as being largely independent of the brain, we now know that these two organs are intricately connected with each other, an insight reflected in the concept of a gut-brain axis. Based on this concept, our digestive system is much more delicate, complex, and powerful than we once assumed. Recent studies suggest that in close interactions with its resident microbes, the gut can influence our basic emotions, our pain sensitivity, and our social interactions, and even guide many of our decisions—and not just those about our food preferences and meal sizes. Validating the popular expression of "gut-based" decision making in neurobiological terms, the complex communication between the gut and the brain plays a role when we make some of our most important life decisions.

The connection between our gut and our mind is not something that solely psychologists should be interested in; it is not just in our heads. The connection is hardwired in the form of anatomical connections between the brain and the gut, and facilitated by biological communication signals carried throughout the bloodstream. But before we get too far, let's take a step back and take a closer look at just what I mean by the "gut"— your digestive system, which is far more complex than a simple food processing machine.

Your gut has capabilities that surpass all your other organs and even rival your brain. It has its own nervous system, known in scientific literature as the enteric nervous system, or ENS, and often referred to in the media as the "second brain." This second brain is made up of 50-100 million nerve cells, as many as are contained in your spinal cord.

The immune cells residing in your gut make up the largest component of your body's immune system; in other words, there are more immune cells living in the wall of your gut than circulating in the blood or residing in your bone marrow. And there is a good reason for the massing of these cells in this particular location, which is exposed to many potentially lethal microorganisms contained in what we eat. The gut-based immune defense system is capable of identifying and destroying a single species of dangerous bacterial invaders that makes it into our digestive system when we accidentally ingest contaminated food or water. What is even more remarkable, it accomplishes this task by recognizing the small number of potentially lethal bacteria in an ocean of a trillion other benevolent microbes living in your gut, the gut microbiota. Accomplishing this challenging task ensures that we can live with our gut microbiota in perfect harmony.

The lining of your gut is studded with a huge number of endocrine cells, specialized cells that contain up to twenty different types of hormones that can be released into the bloodstream if called upon. If you could clump all these endocrine cells together into one mass, it would be greater than all your other endocrine organs—your gonads, thyroid gland, pituitary gland, and adrenal glands—combined.

The gut is also the largest storage facility for serotonin in our body. Ninety-five percent of the body's serotonin is stored in these warehouses. Serotonin is a signaling molecule that plays a crucial role within the gut-brain axis: It is not only essential for normal intestinal functions, such as the coordinated contractions that move food through our digestive system, but it also plays a crucial role in such vital functions as sleep, appetite, pain sensitivity, mood, and overall well-being. Because of the widespread involvement in regulation of some of these brain systems, this signaling molecule is the main target of the major class of antidepressants, the serotonin reuptake inhibitors.

If our gut's sole function was to manage digestion, why would it contain this unparalleled assembly of specialized cells and signaling systems? One answer to this question is a largely unknown feature of our gut, its crucial function as a vast sensory organ, covering the largest surface of our bodies. When spread out, the gut has the size of a basketball court, and it is packed with thousands of little sensors that encode the vast amount of information that is contained in your food in the form of signaling molecules, from sweet to bitter, from hot to cold, and from spicy to soothing.

The gut is connected to the brain through thick nerve cables that can transfer information in both directions and through communication channels that use the bloodstream: hormones and inflammatory signaling molecules produced by the gut signaling up to the brain, and hormones produced by the brain signaling down to the various cells in the gut, such as the smooth muscle, the nerves, and the immune cells, changing their functions. Many of the gut signals reaching the brain will not only generate gut sensations, such as the fullness after a nice meal, nausea and discomfort, and feelings of well-being, but will also trigger responses of the brain that it sends back to the gut, generating distinct gut reactions. And the brain doesn't forget about these feelings, either. Gut feelings are stored in vast databases in the brain, which can later be accessed when making decisions. What we sense in our gut will ultimately affect not only the decisions we make about what to eat and drink, but also the people we choose to spend time with and

FIG. 1. BIDIRECTIONAL COMMUNICATIONS BETWEEN THE GUT AND THE BRAIN

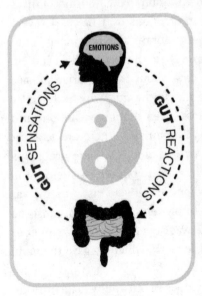

The gut and the brain are closely linked through bidirectional signaling pathways that include nerves, hormones, and inflammatory molecules. Rich sensory information generated in the gut reaches the brain (gut sensations), and the brain sends signals back to the gut to adjust its function (gut reactions). The close interactions of these pathways play a crucial role in the generation of emotions and in optimal gut function. The two are intricately linked.

the way we assess critical information as workers, jury members, and leaders.

In Chinese philosophy, the concept of yin and yang describes how opposite or contrary forces can be viewed as complementary and interconnected, and how they give rise to a unifying whole by interacting with each other. When applied to the brain-gut axis, we can view our gut *feelings* as the yin, and gut *reactions* as the yang. Just as yin and yang are the two complementary principles of the same entity—the brain-gut connection—both the feelings and the reactions are different aspects of the same bidirectional brain-gut network that plays such a crucial role in our well-being, our emotions, and our ability to make intuitive decisions.

The Dawn of the Gut Microbiome

While few people paid much attention to the findings of investigators studying brain-gut interactions over the past several decades, in recent years, the gut-brain axis has taken center stage. This shift can be largely attributed to the exponential rise in knowledge and data about the bacteria, archaea, fungi, and viruses that live inside the gut, which are collectively called the gut microbiota. Even though we are outnumbered by these invisible microorganisms (there are 100,000 times more microbes in your gut alone as there are people on earth), humans only became aware of their existence some three hundred years ago, when Dutch scientist Antonie van Leeuwenhoek made critical improvements to the microscope. When he peered through, he was able to observe live microorganisms from scrapings of the teeth, which he gave the name "animalcules."

Dramatic technological changes in our ability to identify and characterize these microorganisms has occurred since then, and most of this progress has occurred during the past decade. The Human Microbiome Project played a major role in this remarkable progress. The project is an initiative of the U.S. National Institutes of Health launched in October 2007 with the goal of identifying and characterizing the microorganisms living in coexistence with us humans. It was designed to understand the microbial components of our genetic and metabolic landscape, and how they contribute to our normal physiology and disease predisposition.

Over the past decade, the topic of the gut microbiome has spread into virtually every specialty of medicine, even into such widely different specialties as psychiatry and surgery. Invisible communities of microbes are everywhere in our world, including in plants, animals, soils, deep-sea vents, and the upper atmosphere, and as such the fascination with the world of microorganisms also extends to scientists studying microbes inhabiting our oceans, soil, and forests. Even the White House has gotten involved by convening scientists from across the country in 2015 to explore how microbes influence the earth's climate, its food supply, and human health. As of this writing, President Barack Obama plans to announce a national Microbiome Initiative on May 13, 2016, analogous to the earlier Brain Initiative of 2014, which has resulted in billions of dollars of investments into studies of the human brain.

The benefits derived by us humans from our microbiotas have profound consequences for health. Some of the best-documented benefits include assistance in the digestion of food components our guts can't handle by themselves, regulation of our bodies' metabolism, processing and detoxification of dangerous chemicals that we ingest with our food, training and regulation of the immune system, and prevention of invasion and growth of dangerous pathogens. On the other hand,

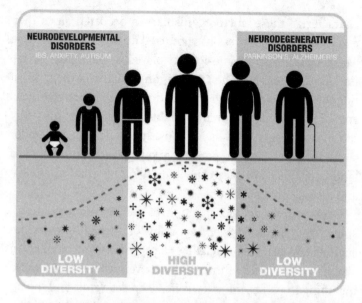

FIG. 2. GUT MICROBIAL DIVERSITY AND VULNERABILITY FOR BRAIN DISORDERS
The diversity and abundance of gut microbes vary over the lifetime of an individual. It is low during the first three years of life when a stable gut microbiome is being established, reaches its maximum during adult life, and decreases as we grow older. The early period of low diversity coincides with the vulnerability window for neurodevelopmental disorders such as autism and anxiety, while the late period of low diversity coincides with the development of neurodegenerative disorders such as Parkinson's and Alzheimer's disease. One may speculate that these low diversity states are risk factors for developing such diseases.

disturbance and alterations in the gut microbiome—gut microbiota and their collective genes and genomes—are associated with a wide variety of diseases, such as inflammatory bowel disease, antibiotic-associated diarrhea, and asthma, and they may even play a role in autism spectrum disorders and neurodegenerative brain disorders like Parkinson's disease.

With the help of new technologies, we're discovering and characterizing distinct microbial populations from our skin, face, nostrils, mouth, lips, eyelids, and even between our teeth. The gastrointestinal tract, in particular the large intestine, however, is home to by far the largest populations. More than 100 trillion microbes live in the dark and nearly oxygen-free world of the human gut—about the same number of all the human cells in the body, if you include the human red blood cells in this comparison. This means that only 10 percent of the cells in or on a human being are actually human. (If you include the body's red blood cells, this number may be closer to 50 percent). If you put all your gut microbes together and shaped them into an organ, it would weigh between 2 and 6 pounds—on par with the brain, which weighs in at 2.6 pounds. Based on this comparison, some people have referred to the gut microbiota as a "forgotten organ." The 1,000 bacterial species that make up the gut microbiota contain more than 7 million genes—or up to 360 bacterial genes for every human gene. This means that less than 1 percent of the combined human and microbial genes (the so-called hologenome) are actually of human origin!

All these genes give the microbes not only an enormous capacity for generating molecules through which they can communicate with us, but also an impressive ability for variation. Gut microbiota differ quite widely from person to person, and no two people's gut microbiota are exactly alike in terms of the many strains and species of microbes they contain. The microbes present in your gut depend on many factors, including your genes, your mother's microbiota, which all of us take on to some extent, the microbes that other members of your household carry, your diet, and—as we will discuss in this book—your brain's activity and state of mind.

To fully grasp the tremendous importance that microbes play in our bodies, it is worth remembering where they came from and how they linked up with us humans. This evolutionary tale has been put into a wonderful narrative by Martin Blaser in his book *Missing Microbes*:

> For about 3 billion years, bacteria were the sole living inhabitants on Earth. They occupied every tranche of land, air and water, driving chemical reactions setting the conditions for the evolution of multicellular life. Slowly, through trial and error across the vastness of time, they invented the complex and robust feedback systems, including the most efficient "language" that to this day supports all life on Earth.

Everything that we've learned about the gut microbiota challenges traditional scientific beliefs, which is one reason why it has become the topic of so much interest and controversy, both in the world of science and the media. It is also the reason why some people are posing deeper, more philosophical questions about the impact of the microbiome: Are our human bodies just a vehicle for the microbes living in it? Do the microbes manipulate our brains to make us seek out foods that are best for *them*? Should the fact that we humans are outnumbered by nonhuman cells change our concept of the human self?

Such philosophical speculations are fascinating, but they are not currently supported by science. However, the implications of what the science of the human microbiome has revealed so far in the last decade are equally profound. And even though we are just at the very beginning of this rapidly unfolding journey of scientific discovery, we can no longer view ourselves as the only intelligent product of evolution, distinct from all the other living creatures on the planet. Just as the Copernican Revolution in the sixteenth century fundamentally changed our understanding of the world's position in the solar system, and Darwin's revolutionary theory of evolution proposed in the nineteenth century has forever changed our position within the animal kingdom, the human microbiome science is forcing us again to reevaluate our position on earth. According to the new science of the microbiome, we humans are truly supraorganisms, composed of closely interconnected human and microbial components, which are inseparable and dependent on each other for survival. And most concerning is the fact that the microbial components are vastly greater than our human contribution to this supraorganism. As the microbial component is so closely connected through a shared biological communication system to all the other microbiomes in the soil, the air, the oceans, and the microbes living in symbiosis with almost all other living creatures, we are closely and inextricably tied into the earth's web of life. The new concept of the human microbial supraorganism clearly has profound implications for our understanding of our role on earth and for many aspects of health and disease.

When the Gut-Microbiota-Brain Axis Falls Out of Balance

The health of any ecosystem can be expressed as its stability and resilience against insults and perturbations. Major factors that contribute to this health are the diversity and abundance of organisms making up the ecosystem. The same considerations apply to our gut microbiome ecosystem. There is growing evidence that the mix of gut microbes falls out of its healthy stable state in several gut disorders (a state called dysbiosis). One of the most serious and best-characterized states of dysbiosis has been reported in a small number of antibiotic-treated hospital patients, who develop severe diarrhea and gut inflammation following the treatment with antibiotics. This so-called *Clostridium difficile* colitis develops when a broad-spectrum antibiotic treatment greatly diminishes the diversity and abundance of the normal gut microbiota, allowing the invasion by the pathogen *C. difficile*. Further confirming the importance of gut microbial diversity for gut health is the observation that the colon inflammation can be rapidly cured by reestablishing the compromised architecture of the gut microbiome. The only currently available way to restore gut microbial diversity in these patients is the transfer of an intact microbiota from the feces of a healthy donor into the gut of the affected patient. This treatment, so-called fecal microbial transplantation, results in an almost miraculous reconstitution of the patient's own microbial composition. We will learn more about this new type of treatment later in this book.

However, the extent and precise role of the dysbiotic state in the pathophysiology of other chronic gut disorders, such as ulcerative colitis, Crohn's disease, or the brain-gut disorder irritable bowel syndrome (IBS), are less completely understood, and many questions remain. Up to 15 percent of the population worldwide suffers from the cardinal IBS symptoms, altered bowel habits, and abdominal pain and discomfort. Several studies have reported altered gut microbial communities in a subset of patients, but it's not clear yet which of the available therapies that aim to restore balance to these gut microbiota (including antibiotics, probiotics, a special diet, or fecal microbial transplantation) work best in individual patients.

The Emerging Role of Microbes

Just a few years ago, it would have sounded like science fiction. But new science confirms that our brains, guts, and gut microbes talk to each other in a shared biological language. How can these invisible creatures talk to us? How can we hear them, and how can they possibly communicate with us?

The microbes not only inhabit the inside of your gut; many of them sit on a razor-thin layer of mucus and cells that coats the inner lining of your intestine. In this unique habitat they are barely separated from the gut's immune cells and the numerous cellular sensors that encode our gut sensations. In other words, they live in intimate contact with the major information-gathering systems in our body. This location allows them to listen in as the brain signals the gut how stressed you are, or when you feel happy, anxious, or angry, even if you are not fully aware of these emotional states. But they do more than just listen. As incredible as this may sound, your gut microbes are in a prime position to influence your emotions, by generating and modulating signals the gut sends back to the brain. Thus, what starts as an emotion in the brain influences your gut and the signals generated by your microbes, and these signals in turn communicate back to the brain, reinforcing and sometimes even prolonging the emotional state.

When the first publications on this topic—mostly animal studies—appeared in the scientific literature some ten years ago, I was skeptical of the results and implications, which just seemed to be too far outside of the conventional view of medicine. However, after my research group at the University of California, Los Angeles, under the leadership of Kirsten Tillisch completed our own study in healthy human subjects, we were able to confirm the results of the animal studies—and I became determined to further explore the question of whether the interactions between the gut microbiota and the brain could affect our background emotions, social interactions, and even our ability to make decisions. Is the proper balance of microbes a prerequisite for mental health? And when these connections between the mind and gut are altered, can they raise a person's risk of developing chronic diseases of the brain? These questions are fascinating not only from a scientist's perspective, but also from a human one: a better understanding of the gut-brain connection is urgently needed in view of the impact that many brain disorders have on human suffering and health care costs.

There has been a dramatic, continuous increase in the reported prevalence of autism spectrum disorders, from 4.5 in 10,000 children in 1966 to 1 in 68 children aged 8 years in 2010. The most recent data from the 2014 National Health Interview reveals that as many as 2.2 percent of U.S. children have received a diagnosis of ASD at some point in their lives, suggesting the current prevalence to be 1 in 58 U.S. children. Some of this increase is likely due to greater awareness and changes in diagnostic criteria, but the evidence also suggests that autism spectrum disorders have become at least twice as prevalent in the last decade alone.

As autism spectrum disorders rose, so did other diseases linked to a change in our gut microbiota, including autoimmune and metabolic disorders. The similarities in the time course of these new epidemics suggested a common underlying mechanism related to a change in our gut microbiota during the last fifty years. Changes in our lifestyles, diet, and in the widespread use of antibiotics have been implicated as possible causes. Recent animal studies have bolstered the link. And recent clinical trials with specific probiotics and with fecal microbial transplantation have begun to directly test the link between gut microbiota and behavioral abnormalities.

Neurodegenerative disorders are on the rise as well. In industrialized countries, one in 100 people over 60 have Parkinson's disease, and in the United States, the disease affects at least half a million people, with about 50,000 new cases diagnosed each year. While it has been estimated that the number of Parkinson's cases will double by 2030, the true prevalence of the disease is difficult to assess, because the disease is typically not diagnosed by its classical neurological signs and symptoms until the disease process is already far advanced. In fact, recent research shows that the enteric nervous system undergoes the nerve degeneration typical of Parkinson's long before classical symptoms of the disease appear, and that changes in patients' gut microbial composition accompany the disease.

Meanwhile, as many as 5 million Americans were living with Alzheimer's disease in 2013, and by 2050, this number is projected to rise nearly threefold to 14 million. Similar to the typical age of onset of Parkinson's, the symptoms of Alzheimer's disease first appear after age 60 and the risk increases with age. The number of people with the disease doubles every 5 years beyond age 65. The economic cost of Alzheimer's is already enormous, and, if present trends continue, it's expected to grow rapidly to $1.1 trillion per year by 2050. Could lifelong alterations in gut microbial function play a role in both of these neurodegenerative disorders, which affect humans at roughly the same age?

Gut microbiota have also been linked to depression, which is the second leading cause of disability in the United States. The drugs used most often to treat depression are the so-called selective serotonin reuptake inhibitors such as Prozac, Paxil, and Celexa. These drugs boost the activity of the serotonin signaling system, which psychiatry had long thought is exclusively located in the brain. However, we know today that 95 percent of the body's serotonin is actually contained in specialized cells in the gut, and these serotonin-containing cells are influenced by what we eat, by chemicals released from certain species of gut microbes, and by signals that the brain sends to them, informing them about our emotional state. What is most remarkable is that these cells are tightly connected to sensory nerves that signal directly back into the brain's emotion regulating centers, making them an important hub within the gut-brain axis. Because of this strategic location it is likely that gut microbes and their metabolites play an important and largely unrecognized role in the development of depression as well as its severity and length—an intriguing possibility that, if confirmed in controlled studies, could create new opportunities for the development of more effective treatments, including specific dietary interventions.

In this book, we will look at new evidence that is beginning to link some of the most devastating brain diseases and some of the most common brain-gut disorders to alterations in how the gut microbes communicate with the brain, and how our lifestyle and diet may impact this connection.

You Are What You Eat—as Long as You Count Your Gut Microbes

"Tell me what you eat, and I will tell you who you are," wrote Jean Anthelme Brillat-Savarin, a French lawyer, physician, and author of an influential nineteenth-century book on the physiology of taste. This connoisseur of high cuisine, for whom Savarin cheese and the Gateau Savarin pastry are named, offered some profound early insights into the relationship between diet, obesity, and indigestion. But back in 1826, when he wrote this, he could not have known that gut microbes mediate how food affects mental well-being and important brain functions. In fact, the gut microbiota residing at the interface between our gut and our nervous system are in a key position to link our physical and mental well-being directly to what we eat and drink, and in turn link our feelings and emotions to the processing of our food.

Your gut gathers information about your food and your environment every millisecond, and it does this twenty-four hours a day, seven days a week, even as you sleep. Much of this information gathering occurs in the stomach and the beginning of the small intestine, where only a small number of microbes reside, and where their contribution to the gut-brain dialogue is likely to be small. But the trillions of microbes living in your large intestine digest remaining food components to produce vast numbers of molecules that add a whole new dimension to this process. As we know from animal experiments, an absence of gut microbes is compatible with life, including the digestion and absorption of nutrients, that is, as long as you live in an environment free of pathogens. However, we now know that such germ-free animals—mice, rats, and even horses— have significant alterations in the development of their brains, in particular in brain regions involved in emotion regulation. Growing up in such a germ-free environment takes a serious toll on the development of your brain.

The well-being of your gut microbes depends on the food you eat, and they are more or less programmed in their food preferences during the first few years in life. However, regardless of their original programming, they can digest virtually everything you feed them, regardless of whether you're an omnivore or a pescatarian. No matter what you feed them, they will use their enormous amount of information stored in their millions of genes to transform partially digested food into hundreds of thousands of metabolites. Even though we are only at the beginning of our understanding what effects these metabolites have on our body, we know that some of them profoundly affect the GI tract, including its nerves and immune cells. Others find their way into the bloodstream and are involved in long-distance signaling, influencing every organ, including the brain. A particularly important role of such microbe-produced molecules is their ability to induce a state of low-grade inflammation in their target organs, which has been implicated in obesity, heart disease, chronic pain, and degenerative diseases of the brain. These inflammatory molecules and their effect on certain brain regions may well be a major clue to our understanding of many human brain disorders.

What Does This New Science Mean for Your Health?

There is no question that the emerging science of gut-brain communication has been one of the most fascinating topics for scientists and the media for the last few years. Who would have ever believed that simply transferring fecal pellets containing gut microbiota from an "extrovert" mouse could change the behavior of a "timid" mouse, making it behave more like the gregarious donor mouse? Or that doing a similar experiment transplanting stool and its microbes from an obese mouse with a voracious appetite would turn a lean mouse into the same overeating animal? Or that the ingestion of a probiotic-enriched yogurt for four weeks in healthy human females could reduce their brains' response to negative emotional stimuli?

The emerging knowledge of an integrated gut microbiota-brain system and its intimate relationship with the food we eat is revealing how the mind, brain, gut, and the gut's microbiota interact. These interactions can either make us vulnerable to a growing number of diseases, or they can help to ensure a state of optimal health. But even more revolutionary, we're now forging a new understanding of disease, health, and mental

well-being, which is based on an ecological view of our bodies, emphasizing the interconnectedness of myriads of players
in the gut and in the brain, creating stability and resistance
against disease.

This new understanding will require us to demand more
from our health care system. We'll need it to move away from
dominant yet outmoded ideas of the body as a complex machine with separate parts, and toward the idea of a highly interconnected ecological system that creates stability and resilience
against disturbances through its diversity. As stated by a famous microbiome scientist, we'll also need it to stop declaring
war on individual cells or microbes and start regarding our gut
microbiome as the friendly park ranger that helps to maintain
biodiversity in a complex ecosystem. This paradigm shift is essential to keep our gut, and therefore our whole selves, healthy
and resilient against disease. This new understanding is likely
to reveal new paths to treat and prevent common diseases that
afflict millions of Americans.

The time has come to empower ourselves to become the
engineers of our own internal ecosystem, and our bodies and
minds. To become your own ecosystem engineer, you will first
need to understand how your brain communicates with your
gut, how your gut communicates with your brain, and how your
gut microbes influence both of these interactions. In the pages
that follow, we will look at the latest scientific findings about
these communication systems. If I'm successful, by the end of
the book you'll be looking at yourself and the world around you
in an entirely new way.

HOW THE MIND COMMUNICATES WITH THE GUT

||||||||||||||||||||||||||||||||||||||||||||||||||||||||||||||||||||||||||||||||||||||||||||||||||||||||||||||||||||||||||||||||||||||||||||||||||||||||||||||||||||||||||||||||

Imagine you're on the freeway, and the driver who's been tailgating you suddenly zips into traffic, swerves abruptly in front of you, and then slams on his brakes. You brake hard to avoid hitting him, causing you to swerve to the next lane. Then you see him laugh. Your neck muscles begin to tense up, your jaw clenches, your lips tighten, your brow furrows. From the passenger seat, your spouse immediately notices your angry expression. In contrast, remember a time when you were depressed. Your face sank, your gaze lowered, and people around you noticed.

Recognizing emotions on other people's faces comes naturally to us. This skill transcends the barriers of language, race, culture, national origin, and even species, as we can recognize an angry dog or a frightened cat. Nature programmed humans to recognize various emotions easily and gauge our responses

accordingly. Your emotions are so apparent because your brain
sends out a distinct pattern of signals to the face's many small
muscles, which means that every emotion has a correspond-
ing facial expression. The people around you can discern your
facial expressions in the blink of an eye. Each of us is an open
book.

But we are literally blind to the gut manifestations of these
emotions. When you are fuming in traffic, your brain sends

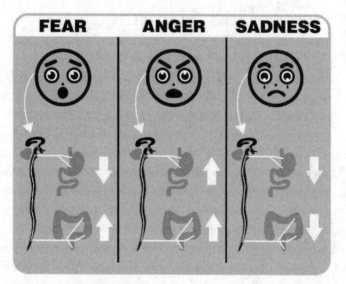

FIG. 3. THE GUT IS A MIRROR IMAGE OF EMOTIONAL FACIAL EXPRESSIONS

*Emotions are closely reflected in a person's facial expressions. A
similar expression of our emotions occurs in the different regions
of the gastrointestinal tract, which is influenced by nerve signals
generated in the limbic system. Signals to the upper and lower
GI tract can be synchronous or go in opposite directions. Solid
white arrows indicate the increase or decrease in gastrointestinal
contractions associated with a particular emotion.*

out a characteristic pattern of signals to your digestive system, just as it does to your facial muscles; the digestive system also responds dramatically. As you sat fuming about the driver who cut you off, your stomach went into vigorous contractions, which increased its production of acid and slowed the emptying of the scrambled eggs you ate for breakfast. Meanwhile your intestines twisted and spit mucus and other digestive juices. A similar yet distinct pattern happens when you're anxious or upset. When you're depressed, your intestines hardly move at all. In fact, we now know that your gut mirrors every emotion that arises in your brain.

The activity of these brain circuits affects other organs as well, creating a coordinated response to every emotion you feel. When you're stressed, for example, your heartbeat speeds and your neck and shoulder muscles tighten, and the reverse happens when you're relaxed. But the brain is tied to the gut like no other organ, with far more extensive, hardwired connections. Because people have always felt emotion in their gut, our language is rich with expressions that reflect this. Every time your stomach was tied up in knots, you had a gut-wrenching experience, or you felt butterflies in your stomach, it was the emotion-generating circuits of your brain that were responsible. Your emotions, brain, and gut are uniquely connected.

If a patient with abnormal gut reactions seeks help from the medical system and an endoscopy does not reveal something more serious, such as gut inflammation or a tumor, physicians often dismiss the importance of the patient's symptoms. Frustrated about their inability to provide effective relief, they tend to recommend special diets, probiotics, or pills to normalize abnormal bowel habits, without addressing the true cause of the gut reaction.

If more doctors and patients realized that the gut is in fact a theater in which the drama of emotion plays out, that drama might be less likely to become a painful melodrama for patients. Nearly 15 percent of the U.S. population suffers from a range of aberrant gut reactions, including irritable bowel syndrome, chronic constipation, indigestion, and functional heartburn, which all fall into the category of brain-gut disorders. They suffer from symptoms that range from queasiness, gurgling, and bloating all the way to unbearable pain. Amazingly, the majority of patients suffering from abnormal gut reactions have no idea that their gut problems reflect their emotional state.

Even more amazingly, most of the time neither do their doctors.

The Man Who Could Not Stop Vomiting

Of the many patients I have seen in my long career as a gastroenterologist, Bill stands out in my memory more than any other. Bill was twenty-five and otherwise healthy when he came to my office with his fifty-two-year-old mother. Surprisingly, it was she who started the conversation: "I really hope you can help Bill. You are our last resort. We are desperate."

Over the previous eight years, Bill had spent countless hours in various emergency rooms, suffering from excruciating stomach pain and unstoppable vomiting. During particularly difficult periods, he would visit the ER several times a week. Usually the ER physicians prescribed painkillers and sedatives to treat his discomfort, but none of them seemed to have any idea what was actually wrong with him. Even worse, some labeled him a drug-seeking patient because nothing in the diagnostic tests they ran matched the severity of his symptoms.

Bill had also been to several gastrointestinal (GI) specialists who performed extensive diagnostic tests but without finding a cause for his miserable symptoms. His continued pain and vomiting forced him to drop out of college and move back in with his concerned parents.

His mother, a businesswoman, was frustrated that Bill's doctors had not been able to diagnose Bill accurately, so she began searching online for answers. "I think he has all the symptoms of cyclical vomiting syndrome," she told me.

As Bill's doctor, I wanted to see for myself.

As happens often with brain-gut disorders, many unusual theories have been proposed to explain the unique constellation of symptoms in cyclical vomiting syndrome. But based on decades of research that my team has done with several other research groups at UCLA, I believed that the most plausible explanation was an exaggerated gut reaction triggered by an overactive stress response in the brain.

In patients with cyclical vomiting syndrome, stressful life events generally spark the attacks. A wide range of seemingly unrelated stimuli including strenuous exercise, menstruation, exposure to high altitudes, or simple prolonged psychological stress can cause enough of an imbalance in the body to trigger an attack. When the brain (not necessarily our conscious brain) perceives such a threat, it signals the hypothalamus, an important brain region coordinating all our vital functions, to crank up release of a critical stress molecule called corticotropin-releasing factor, or CRF for short, which functions as a master switch that sends the brain (and the body) into stress-response mode. Patients with this disorder may be completely symptom-free for several months or even years, even though their CRF system is primed all the time. But when they experience additional stress, a recurrence of symptoms is triggered.

When CRF levels rise high enough, it switches every organ and cell in your body, including the gut, into stress mode. In a series of elegant animal experiments, my UCLA colleague Yvette Tache, who's one of the world's experts in stress-induced brain-gut interactions, revealed the many shifts in the body that CRF induces.

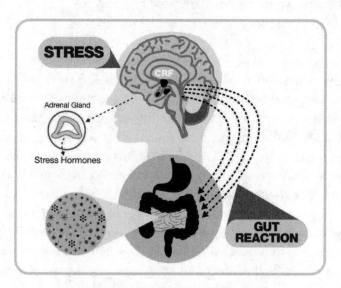

FIG. 4. GUT REACTIONS IN RESPONSE TO STRESS

In response to any perturbations of an individual's normal balanced state such as stress, the brain mounts a coordinated response aimed at optimizing the organism's well-being and survival. The corticotropin releasing factor (CRF) is the chemical master switch that sets this stress response in motion. It is secreted by the hypothalamus and acts on closely adjacent regions of the brain. Stress-induced CRF in the brain is associated with an increase in stress hormones (such as cortisol and norepinephrine) in the body. This process also stimulates a stress-induced gut reaction that impacts the composition and activity of the gut microbiota.

In the brain, spiking CRF levels raise anxiety and make people more sensitive to a range of sensations, including signals from the gut, which are experienced as severe belly pain. The gut itself contracts more and its contents are evacuated, resulting in diarrhea. The stomach slows down and even reverses itself to empty its contents upward. The gut wall becomes leakier, the colon secretes more water and mucus, and the amount of blood flowing through the lining of our stomach and intestine increases.

In Bill's case, just a few key questions about his symptoms would help me make a diagnosis. I asked Bill if he was completely symptom-free in between his bouts of vomiting, which was the case. I asked him and his mother whether there was a family history of migraine headaches, a chronic pain disorder genetically related to cyclical vomiting syndrome. And indeed, both his mother and grandmother suffered from migraines.

"What kind of symptoms do you experience in the period immediately before an attack?" I asked. Bill told me that a full-blown attack was usually preceded by about fifteen minutes of intense anxiety, sweating, cold hands, and pounding of his heart—all symptoms of a stresslike reaction in his body. What's more, these symptoms woke him up very early in the morning—another identifying feature of the syndrome. (This feature is probably caused by the diurnal increase in the activity of our central stress system.) A hot shower or an Ativan pill could prevent the attacks, but most of the time that didn't help. "Once the vomiting begins, and I can't stop it, I have to rush to the emergency room."

"What happens in the emergency room?" I asked. Bill told me that his doctors reluctantly gave him narcotic painkillers, which usually put him right to sleep, and he'd wake up symptom-free an hour later. Bill's many previous diagnostic tests, including endoscopies and CT scans of his belly, had not revealed any abnormalities that could explain his symptoms, and a brain scan had ruled out a brain tumor.

Bill's mother's Internet diagnosis was indeed correct—he was suffering from cyclical vomiting syndrome. The sad thing was that despite his doctors' repeated failure to diagnose him correctly, making the correct diagnosis was actually simple, and his mother, who had no medical training, did it on the Internet.

You don't have to suffer from the crippling symptoms of cyclical vomiting syndrome to experience the limited knowledge that many physicians have about gut reactions gone wrong, and the resulting lack of effective therapies. Nearly 3 in 20 people in the United States suffer from symptoms or syndromes caused by problems from altered brain-gut interactions, including irritable bowel syndrome, functional heartburn, or functional dyspepsia. However, those of you who are not bothered by nasty and unpleasant gut sensations should be aware that you don't have to have any of these disorders for gut reactions to occur.

Cyclical vomiting syndrome is one of the most dramatic examples of gut reactions gone awry, but it is not the only one. Altered brain-gut interactions can have powerful effects on all of us.

The Little Brain in Your Gut

Imagine that you're out to dinner with a good friend. The waiter has just served you a medium-rare ribeye and you are reveling in the deliciousness of the meal. Here is a short account of what happens the minute you put the first piece of steak in your mouth—though you may want to avoid making what follows a part of your dinner conversation.

Even before you chew and swallow your food, your stomach

fills with concentrated hydrochloric acid that can be as acidic as battery acid. When the partially chewed bites of steak get there, your stomach exerts grinding forces so intense that they break up the steak into tiny particles.

Meanwhile, your gallbladder and pancreas are preparing the small intestine to do its job, by injecting bile to help digest fat, and a variety of digestive enzymes. When your stomach passes the tiny steak particles to the small intestine, the enzymes and bile break them down into nutrients that the gut can absorb and transfer to the rest of the body.

As digestion proceeds, the muscles in your intestinal walls execute a distinct pattern of muscular contractions called peristalsis, which moves food down and through your digestive tract. The strength, length, and direction of peristalsis depend on the type of food you have ingested, ensuring, for example, that the gut has more time to absorb fat and complex carbohydrates, and less for a sugary drink.

At the same time, parts of your intestinal walls contract to steer the food being digested to the lining of the small intestine, where nutrients are absorbed. In your large intestine, powerful waves of contraction move contents back and forth to enable the organ to extract and absorb 90 percent of the water in intestinal contents. Another powerful wave of contraction then moves contents toward the rectum, typically triggering an urge to have a bowel movement.

Between meals, a different pressure wave—the migrating motor complex—serves as your gut's housekeeper, sweeping out anything else your stomach couldn't dissolve or break down into small enough pieces such as undissolved medications and unchewed peanuts. This wave slowly travels from the esophagus to your rectum every ninety minutes, generating enough pressure to crack a Brazil nut and sweeping undesirable microbes from your small intestine into the colon.

Unlike the peristaltic reflex, this housekeeping wave operates only when there's no food left to digest in your GI tract—when you're sleeping, for example—and it switches off as soon you take your first bite of breakfast.

The gut can coordinate all this and more without any help from your brain or spinal cord, and it is not the muscles making up your gut wall that know how to do it. Instead, managing digestion is largely the work of your enteric nervous system (ENS)—a remarkable network of 50 million nerve cells wrapped around the intestine from the esophagus to the rectum. This "second brain" may be smaller than its three-pound counterpart in your head, but when it comes to digestion, it's brilliant.

Michael Gershon, a prominent anatomist and cell biologist at Columbia University Medical Center, a pioneer in studying the role of the gut's serotonin system, and author of the popular book *The Second Brain*, likes to show a video clip that demonstrates the enteric nervous system's ability to operate independently. In it, a section of guinea pig intestine sits in a bath of fluid, and on its own propels a plastic pellet from one side of the intestine to the other—all without any connection to the brain. In all likelihood, the human gut can operate just as independently.

It's remarkable that all of these complex digestive functions are coordinated autonomously by hardwired circuits—anatomic connections between millions of nerve cells—within your enteric nervous system, and that this is accomplished without much help from your brain or the rest of your central nervous system—as long as everything goes well.

On the other hand, your emotional brain can mess up just about every one of those seemingly automatic functions. If your dinner conversation takes a wrong turn and you get into an argument with your friend, your stomach's wonderful meat-grinding activity is quickly turned off and instead goes into spastic contractions that no longer allow it to empty properly. Half of that tasty steak you ate will remain in your stomach without further digestion. Long after you have left the restaurant, your stomach will still be in spasms as you lie awake. Because there is still food in your stomach, the nocturnal migrating contractions won't happen, preventing the usual overnight cleansing of your gut. In patients like Bill, who have a hyperactive brain-gut axis to start out with, stress-related or emotional triggers that won't cause much harm to a healthy individual will forcefully inhibit stomach peristalsis and even reverse it, while at the same time creating spastic contractions in his colon. It is as if the set points on the warning system in his brain are off, triggering frequent false alarms, with devastating consequences for his well-being.

Gunshots and Gut Reactions

Humans have always experienced emotion via their guts, and over the years, many curious individuals have tried to learn more about this phenomenon. When army surgeon William Beaumont was presented with the opportunity to learn more about the gut-brain connection in 1822, he didn't hesitate.

It was early summer, and Beaumont was stationed at Fort Mackinac on Mackinac Island, Michigan, in the upper reaches of Lake Huron. A fur trapper named Alexis St. Martin had been accidentally shot with a musket from less than a yard away. When Dr. Beaumont first saw him a half hour after the accident, St. Martin had a hole the size of a man's hand in his upper left abdomen. Looking into the wound, Beaumont could see the man's stomach, which had a hole large enough to fit an index finger.

Beaumont's excellent surgical care saved St. Martin's life, but he wasn't able to close the man's stomach wound, and St. Martin ended up with a gastric fistula—a permanent hole in his stomach that opened to the outside of his body. After St. Martin recovered, he was no longer able do the physical work of a fur trader, so when Beaumont relocated from Michigan to Fort Niagara in New York State, he hired St. Martin to work with his family as a live-in handyman, and the two became an unusual team of investigator and study subject.

Before long, Beaumont became the first person in history to observe human digestion in real time. He conducted an experiment with St. Martin in which he tied small pieces of boiled beef, raw cabbage, stale bread, and other foods to a silk string and then dangled them in St. Martin's stomach, pulling them out at different times to test how "gastric juice" from the stomach digested food. The experiments were difficult and uncomfortable for St. Martin, who sometimes became upset and irritable. By directly observing the changes that occurred in St. Martin's gastric activity, Beaumont concluded that the man's anger slowed his digestion. In this way, Beaumont became the first scientist in history to report that your emotions can influence the activity of your stomach.

Emotions impact not just the stomach, but your entire digestive tract. As reported by Weeks in 1946, an army physician working in a field during World War II observed a wounded soldier who had suffered extensive combat-related damage to the wall of his abdomen, exposing large portions of his small and large intestine. Doctors observed that when this unfortunate soldier's injured compatriots began to arrive in the same hospital ward, causing the wounded soldier even more distress, the movement in both his small and large intestine became more active.

It took some twenty years from these graphic early wartime

observations to more scientific laboratory studies of mind-gut connections. In the 1960s, an accomplished gastroenterologist at Dartmouth College's school of medicine, Thomas Almy, examined a larger number of patients under more controlled conditions. He conducted emotionally charged interviews with healthy people and patients with irritable bowel syndrome and monitored the colonic activity of both groups. When subjects reacted with hostility and aggression, their colons contracted quickly, whereas when they felt hopeless, inadequate, or self-reproaching, their colons contracted more slowly. Later, other scientists confirmed these results and found that colonic activity was increased only when topics discussed were personally relevant to the subjects.

Today, scientists agree that the brain is hardwired to link the emotions you experience every day with specific bodily responses. And when push comes to shove, hardwiring directs our gut reactions.

Here is an analogy that I like to use with my patients to help them understand how the brain, enteric nervous system, and gut interact.

Imagine that a hurricane is approaching. The federal government doesn't send emergency instructions to every individual citizen in the country. Instead, it sends instructions to a network of local agencies, which can broadcast and implement the plans if needed. In the absence of a major threat like a natural disaster, these local agencies can regulate most everything on their own. But when a clear directive comes down from the federal government during an emergency, it overrides many routine activities going on at the local level. Once the threat has passed, the country returns quickly to its regular activities.

Similarly, your enteric nervous system can handle all routine challenges related to digestion. However, when you perceive a threat and feel afraid or angry, the emotional brain center does not send individual instructions to every single cell in the gastrointestinal tract. Instead, the brain's emotional circuits signal the enteric nervous system to divert from its daily routine. The digestive system switches back to local control once the emotion has passed.

Your brain implements these motor programs in the gut through a variety of mechanisms. It releases stress hormones such as cortisol and adrenaline (also known as epinephrine) and dispatches nerve signals to the enteric nervous system. The brain sends two sets of nerve signals: those that stimulate (carried by the parasympathetic nerves, including the vagus nerve) and those that inhibit gut function (the sympathetic nerves). Usually activated in tandem, the two nerve pathways do a remarkable job of adjusting, fine-tuning, and coordinating the activities of the enteric nervous system to shape gut activity reflecting a particular emotion.

When your emotions play out in the theater of your gut, a large ensemble of specialized cells are at work. The actors include various types of gut cells, cells of the enteric nervous system, and the gut's 100 trillion microbes—and the play's emotional overtones will alter their behavior and their chemical conversations. The plots rotate throughout your day, and include both negative and positive stories. On the one hand, there are worries about your children; irritation when the guy in the next lane cuts you off on the highway; anxiety when you're running late to the meeting; fear of layoffs and financial stress.

On the other, there's also a hug from your spouse, kind words from a friend, or a pleasant family meal. While we have learned a lot about the gut reactions associated with such negative emotions as anger, sorrow, and fear, we know virtually nothing about the gut reactions to positive emotions such as love, bonding, and happiness. Does the brain refrain from in-terfering with the activities of the enteric nervous system when everything is fine? Or does it send a distinct set of nerve sig-nals that reflect your state of happiness? And what effect would such happy signals have on the gut microbes, on gut sensitiv-ity, and on the digestion of a meal? What happens in your gut when you sit down for a meal with your family to celebrate the graduation of your daughter from college, or when you are in a blissful state during a meditation retreat? These are important questions that science will need to answer if we want to fully grasp the impact of gut reactions on our well-being.

For some people, the plays performed in the gut include more thrillers and horror stories than romantic comedies. Gut cells in a chronically angry or anxious person, using a script that dates back to childhood, may play out dark plots day after day. Many gut cells in these people over time adapt to accommodate the stage directions: nerve connections in the enteric nervous system change, the sensors in the gut become more sensitive, the gut's serotonin-producing machinery shifts into higher gear, and even gut microbes become more aggressive. It's no surprise that when scientists study the gut in patients with functional GI disorders, anxiety disorders, depression, or au-tism, they find changes in the makeup and behavior of many of these gut players, and the scientific literature is filled with such observations. However, developing therapies targeted at such gut changes has generally failed to provide symptomatic relief for patients with these disorders. On the other hand, one would expect that changing the playbook of the brain to more positive stories, with the goal of altering the gut reactions and thereby reversing the cellular changes in the gut, is more promising. Studies are currently under way to determine if gut microbial changes are associated with positive mind-based interventions, such as hypnosis and meditation, and if these changes lead to symptom improvements in such disorders as irritable bowel syndrome.

How the Brain Programs the Gut's Emotional Responses

Today, we know a great deal about how emotion affects our bodies, including our GI tract. To understand how it works, you first need to know about the limbic system, a primitive brain system that we share with other warm-blooded animals and that plays a major role generating your emotions. Deep in your gray matter, emotion-specific circuits within the limbic system get activated when you're angry, scared, feel sexually attracted, or hurt—and also when you feel hungry or thirsty.

Like a miniature supercomputer, these circuits aim to adjust our bodies to respond optimally to changes both inside and outside our bodies. When we face a life-threatening situation, it can turn on a dime, quickly rearranging thousands of messages to individual cells and organs throughout the body, which shift their behavior just as quickly.

We're all familiar with what happens next. The emotion-related brain circuits send signals to the stomach and intestine to rid themselves of contents that might otherwise drain energy required for action, which is why you might need to head to the bathroom before your big presentation. Our cardiovascular system reroutes oxygen-rich blood from the gut to the muscles, slowing digestion and preparing us to fight (or flee).

We're not alone in the animal kingdom in these experiences: For millions of years, mammals have needed to bond, fight,

assess potential threats, and sometimes flee. Evolution has be-
stowed upon us a collective wisdom about how to best respond
to these situations, and has packaged that wisdom into specific
circuits and programs that execute our reactions to threats automatically. This saves time and energy in a moment of crisis
because without such hardwired responses, we'd have to start
from scratch each time. These programs, known as emotional
operating programs, can activate within milliseconds, implementing a coordinated set of behaviors that allow us to survive,
thrive, and reproduce.

Jaak Panksepp, a neuroscientist at Washington State University who has made important contributions to the field of affective neuroscience (which applies neuroscience to the study of
emotion), has concluded from his experiments on animals that
our brains have at least seven emotional operating programs
that direct the body's response to fear, anger, sorrow, play, lust,
love, and maternal nurturance. They execute the appropriate
set of bodily responses quickly and automatically—even when
you don't know you're feeling a particular emotion. They make
your face flush when you feel embarrassed, give you goose
bumps when you watch a scary movie, make your heart beat
faster when you're scared, and make your gut more sensitive
when you are worried.

Our emotional operating programs are written in our genes.
This genetic coding is, in part, inherited from our parents, and
it is also influenced by events we experience early in life. For
example, you may have inherited genes that predispose your
fear or anger program to overreact to stressful situations. If
you also experienced emotional trauma as a child, your body
added chemical tags to these key stress-response genes. The
net result is that as an adult, you will most likely experience
exaggerated gut reactions to stress. This explains the common
observation that two individuals exposed to the same stressful

situation may show very different reactions to it: while one does not experience any noticeable gut reaction, the other one is incapacitated by nausea, stomach cramps, and diarrhea. While this early programming for trouble may be a good thing for surviving in a dangerous world, it is a liability if you live in the safety of a protected environment.

When the Gut Gets Stressed

Of all of our emotional operating programs, the one engaged by stressful events is among the best studied. When you feel anxious or fearful, your stress response is at work, trying to maintain a state of homeostasis, or internal balance, in the face of internal or external threats.

When we talk about stress, we usually talk about stress from daily living pressures, or larger stressors such as trauma or natural disasters. But your brain also perceives many bodily events as stressful, including infections, surgeries, accidents, food poisoning, sleep deficits, attempts to stop smoking, or even something as natural as a woman's menstrual period.

Let's pull back the curtain on what happens in your body when you're stressed. But first, you need to know more about the emotional brain's impressive abilities. Life-threatening situations showcase them best.

If the brain decides there's a threat, it activates the stress program in the brain, which then orchestrates the most appropriate response in our bodies, including the gastrointestinal tract. Each of our emotional operating programs uses a specific signaling molecule, so the release of a particular substance in the brain can trigger the engagement of the entire program with all its consequences on the body and the gut. The brain's dedicated signaling molecules include a few hormones you've probably heard about before—endorphins, which act as a painkiller in the body and promotes a feeling of well-being; dopamine, which triggers desire and motivation; and oxytocin, which is sometimes called the "love hormone" and stimulates feelings of trust and attraction. They also include the molecule mentioned earlier known as corticotropin-releasing factor, or CRF, which acts as the stress master switch.

Even if you're perfectly healthy and relaxing on a beach, CRF plays a crucial role for your well-being by regulating the amount of the hormone cortisol that is produced by your adrenal glands. Through its normal daily fluctuations, cortisol maintains proper fat, protein, and carbohydrate metabolism and helps keep the immune system in check.

However, when the stress program is activated, there is a dramatic increase in this CRF-cortisol system. When you are stressed, the first responder in your brain is the hypothalamus, a small brain region that controls all your vital functions and is the main production site for CRF. Through a chemical intermediary, the CRF release is followed by activation of the adrenal gland, which starts pumping out cortisol, thereby increasing its level in the bloodstream and preparing the body for the expected increased metabolic demand.

As the stress master switch, CRF released from the hypothalamus also spreads locally to another brain region, the amygdala, which triggers a feeling of anxiety or even fear. This activation of the amygdala plays out in the body as heart palpitations, sweaty palms, and the urge to eliminate any contents from the GI tract.

These stress-induced changes in your digestive system may not sound like the ideal way to enjoy a meal, and they're not. The next time you're in the midst of a particularly stressful day, just remember that you might not want to eat a large lunch.

Even if you eat when you're more relaxed, there's still a

chance you could experience an unpleasant gut reaction to your meal. Once an emotional motor program has been triggered, its effects may linger for hours—or sometimes for years. Our thoughts, memories of past events, and expectations of the future can influence the activities within our brain-gut axis, and the consequences can sometimes be painful.

For example, if you return to the restaurant where you argued with your spouse over dinner, your memories may trigger your anger operating program, despite a friendly dinner conversation this time around. If that restaurant was an Italian restaurant, any Italian restaurant or even the mere thought of risotto di mare may trigger the anger program. I often explain this scenario to my patients, who are quick to blame certain foods for causing digestive distress. I ask them to explore whether it's the food or in fact a recollection of an earlier event that's responsible for their symptoms. When they start paying attention to the circumstances that trigger their symptoms, they often realize the incredible power of the brain-gut connection.

The Mirror in Your Gut

One of the most important pieces of information I can give to a patient like Bill, with cyclical vomiting syndrome, or to patients with other disorders of the brain-gut axis, is a simple, scientific explanation of what causes their distressing symptoms, and how this information determines the treatment of this condition. This simple explanation generally relieves the uncertainty about the diagnosis, which tends to ease the patient's mind as well as the family's. Science also forms the rational basis for tailoring an effective therapy.

In the clinic, I told Bill that his brain was releasing too much CRF. Excess CRF in his brain was prompting not just his feeling of anxiety, but also the associated heart palpitations, sweaty palms, exaggerated stomach contractions that reversed peristalsis and sent his stomach contents upward, and excessive contractions of his colon, which were associated with cramping pain and sent his stomach contents downward. Bill and his mother were visibly relieved by the information, as it was apparently the first time that anyone had given them a scientific explanation for his symptoms.

"But why do the attacks always happen in the early morning hours?" Bill's mother wanted to know. I told her that the normal secretion of CRF in the brain naturally peaks in the early morning hours, and gradually declines until midday. So in patients with cyclical vomiting syndrome, brain CRF would most likely reach unhealthy levels early in the morning.

I told them about how CRF declares an emergency and shifts the body from peacetime to war, to teach them how our brain and our gut's nervous system work together to direct gut function. "This makes total sense," Bill said, "but why does it happen in my case without any major stresses in the middle of my sleep?"

"That's exactly where the problem is," I responded, explaining how the normal brakes on his brain's emergency mechanisms were faulty, which caused trivial events to trigger his fear-related program. "This will result in many false alarms," I said.

"I am so glad that we finally know what's going on," said his mother. But an explanation only gets you halfway to a solution. She asked what they could do to prevent the attacks from happening in the first place.

To help Bill prevent the vicious attacks that were keeping him from living a full life, I prescribed several medications that calm hyperactive stress circuits and the hyperarousal associated with the excessive CRF release. Some of these aimed to reduce the frequency of his attacks, others to stop an attack in its tracks should one occur. Fortunately, with proper treatment, most cyclical vomiting patients improve dramatically—they have fewer attacks, and they get better at stopping a developing attack. Over time, patients lose the fear of recurring attacks that had held them back, which often allows them to reduce or discontinue the medication.

This was exactly what happened with Bill. When I saw him three months later, he had only had a single episode, and he had stopped it by taking Klonopin, an antianxiety medication I had prescribed. After years of suffering and enduring humiliating comments from emergency room physicians, he was excited to finally be able to rebuild his life. Other cyclical vomiting patients I've seen have required additional treatments to recover, including cognitive behavioral therapy and hypnosis. But Bill did not. He resumed his college classes and was even able to greatly reduce his medication over time.

We can all learn from patients like Bill, as I do every day in the clinic. Normal gut reactions, such as worrying about a job interview, or transient upsets from being stuck in traffic or running late to an appointment are never a major problem. However, we should be mindful of the detrimental effects of such emotions on our gut and its many residents when they occur chronically, in the form of anger, sorrow, or recurrent fear. Remember, the stage on which these gut reactions play out is large, and the number of actors is huge. This may not be such a big deal in the case of a feeling of thirst, which we can easily quench with a glass of water, or an acute pain that only lasts a few minutes. It is of greater concern when we recall that emotions always have a mirror image in our gut, and speculate about the detrimental effects that chronic anger, sorrow, or fear may exert not only on our digestive health but on our overall well-being.

CHAPTER

3

HOW YOUR GUT TALKS
TO YOUR BRAIN

From morning to night, as you wrestle with the responsibilities of everyday life, how often do you think about what's happening in your belly? If you're like most people, probably not much. But as quietly as our guts usually go about their business, the events in your stomach and intestines are momentous. To get a firsthand impression of these gut sensations, try this experiment: take a day when you're not too distracted, and focus your attention from morning to night on all the sensations that your gut generates throughout the day.

These are the sensations you normally wouldn't pay much attention to—the subtle physical feelings and sounds, as well as the background emotions that accompany them. Try to be mindful of as many of these sensations as you can, and write them down on a sheet of paper or dictate them into your smartphone as they occur. You may also want to add information about what you were doing at the time, how you were feeling, and what you were eating. Here is an example of such an experiment—one day's worth of gut sensations performed by Judy, a healthy, twenty-six-year-old research volunteer who participated in a study we conducted many years ago.

Judy wakes up early on Sunday morning, has a cup of coffee, then goes on her daily morning run. She doesn't eat anything before the three-mile run because she knows from experience that running on a full stomach interferes with her exercise. When she returns from her run, she makes her weekly phone calls to her mother and to a good friend. By the time she's done speaking with them, she is starving and craving her usual Sunday breakfast—a mushroom omelet and a fresh sourdough baguette with cream cheese.

She enjoys the breakfast, getting a pleasant feeling from savoring this favorite meal. At the same time, she doesn't pay that much attention to what she's eating because she is reading an interesting article in the newspaper. At some point she feels full and leaves half of the uneaten omelet on her plate. She has made plans to go bicycling at the beach with her boyfriend, and before she leaves the house, she needs to go to the bathroom for a bowel movement. She and her boyfriend have a great time at the beach. When she gets back home, it's 7 p.m.

After having a light dinner, Judy realizes that she hasn't spent any time on a work presentation she has to give on Monday morning. She starts worrying, and notices a queasy feeling in the pit of her stomach. The feeling slowly improves as she tries to finish her presentation and at 10 p.m., she decides to go to bed and get up early the next morning to perfect the presentation. She sets her alarm clock for 5:30 a.m. but doesn't sleep well. Each time she wakes up, she notices a gurgling sensation in her belly; sometimes it feels like a long, loud rumbling that slowly migrates down the length of her abdomen. She finally gets up, goes to the kitchen, and finishes the leftover omelet from breakfast. The rumbling noises stop, and she feels better and goes back to sleep.

When you think about it, you likely experience similar gut sensations on a daily basis, although you may not be fully aware of them. We've all lived with these sensations our entire lives, and they have become second nature. From the perspective of sheer survival, this general lack of attention to and awareness of our gut sensations is a good thing: Navigating the complexities and information overflow of the modern world is hard enough already. Can you imagine spending each day focused on the rumblings and contractions of your gut, or being forced awake every evening when another wave of high-amplitude contractions sweeps through your GI tract? If we had to continuously attend to these sensations we wouldn't be able to concentrate on anything else. You wouldn't be able to carry on a dinner conversation, take a nap after lunch, read the *New York Times* Sunday edition, or sleep through the night.

The only gut sensations that we are generally aware of are those that require a response: a sensation of hunger that prompts us to eat something, a sensation of satiety when it is time to stop eating, or a sensation of fullness in our belly that makes us look for a toilet. We remain blissfully unaware of most gut sensations until we experience some gastro-calamity such as a stomachache, heartburn, nausea, a persistent sense of bloating, or, worse, a bout of food poisoning or a viral gastroenteritis. Or we may just feel we ate too much and feel awful, even after eating a normal-sized meal. Suddenly the sensory information from our gut becomes quite relevant—and usually for good reasons. These unpleasant sensations drive us to seek help, and they help us avoid whatever caused our distress in the future by making sure we never forget.

The Brain That Felt Too Much

While most people are consciously unaware of virtually all their gut sensations, there are some notable exceptions. One involves the very select group of people who are easily able to feel their heartbeats and food moving through their intestines. These individuals show an increased awareness of all signals from their bodies, including those arising from the gut. In brain imaging experiments, they have been shown to have heightened responses of brain networks that are concerned with attention and salience assessment.

The other exceptions to this rule are the unfortunate 10 percent of the population who perceive corrupted signals from their gut that don't match the actual sensory information transmitted to the brain. Out of the many patients I have seen in my practice, one very pleasant gentleman stands out in terms of his unique history, which illustrates this concept of increased awareness of bodily sensations.

Frank was a seventy-five-year-old retired schoolteacher who came to see me with GI problems he had been experiencing over the last five years, including typical IBS symptoms of abdominal bloating and discomfort, and irregular bowel movements. However, the IBS symptoms were not his only problem. He also experienced a chronic, unpleasant sensation that felt as if something were stuck in the upper part of his esophagus (so called globus sensation), frequent episodes of belching, sensations of discomfort behind his sternum (his chest bone) that sometimes had a menthol-like quality and made him cough, and the sensation of not getting enough air when taking a breath. These symptoms started suddenly about five years before he came to see me. The onset of his symptoms coincided with the loss of his wife due to a serious illness.

When I pressed for more information that would help me make a diagnosis, Frank admitted that he had been experiencing mild IBS like symptoms since childhood. As Frank had undergone repeated extensive diagnostic evaluations of his chest, his gastrointestinal tract, and his heart, which did not reveal any plausible cause for his symptoms, it seemed most likely that he was suffering from some sort of functional gastrointestinal disorder. His symptoms were most consistent with a generalized hypersensitivity to gut sensations coming from different regions of his gastrointestinal tract, from the beginning of his esophagus all the way to the end of his colon. While some physicians might dismiss his symptoms as purely psychological in nature, we now know that there is an elaborate sensory machinery located in our gastrointestinal tract, including the specialized molecules (so-called receptors) that can recognize different chemicals including menthol. But what could have triggered this hypersensitivity in Frank five years ago?

Frank's partner provided one potential explanation: Frank had long been eating an unhealthy diet, including foods high in animal fats and sugar. She had noticed that his symptoms got worse when he couldn't control his craving for chocolate cake, pizza, french fries, or rich cheeses. Is it possible that these high-fat food items may have played a role in the sensitization of his gut-brain communication? Patients like Frank are not only more sensitive to normal gut functions, such as contractions, distensions, and acid secretion. We know from many studies in patients like Frank that some of them are also more sensitive to experimental stimuli such as inflating a balloon in their intestine, or exposing their esophagus to an acidic solution.

Given the complexity of the gut's sensory system, it is no surprise that this system is vulnerable to disturbances, like overreacting to normal food components, or being hypersensitive to food additives or changes in food supply that may not be good for us, but which are tolerated by the majority of people without any symptoms. Could it be that people like Frank are the canaries in the coal mine, the first to be affected by some pending calamity?

More than 90 percent of the sensory information collected by your gut never reaches conscious awareness. For most of us it's easy to ignore the daily sensations from our belly; yet the enteric nervous system is monitoring them very carefully. Through a complex system of sensory mechanisms, many of your gut sensations are quietly directed to the little brain in your gut, providing it with vital information to ensure optimal functioning of your digestive system twenty-four hours a day. But a huge flow of gut sensations is also directed upward, to the brain. Ninety percent of the signals conveyed through the vagus nerve travel from the gut to the brain, while just 10 percent of the traffic runs in the opposite direction, from the brain to the gut. In fact, the gut can handle most of its activities without any interference from the brain, while the brain seems to depend greatly on vital information from the gut.

What information is your gut reporting on that's so vital? Far more than you might imagine. The many sensors in your gut inform the enteric nervous system about everything it needs to know in order to generate the most appropriate pattern of contractions, that is, the strength and direction of the gut's peristalsis to speed or slow the transit of ingested food through the stomach and intestine, and to produce the right amount of acid and bile to ensure proper digestion. It gathers information pertaining to the presence and amount of food in the stomach, the size and consistency of the food you swallow, the chemical composition of an ingested meal, and even the presence and activity of your community of gut microbiota. In case of an emergency, these sensors will also detect the presence of parasites, viruses, or pathogenic bacteria, or their toxins, as well as the gut's inflammatory response. In fact, acute gut inflammation will make many of the sensors more sensitive to normal stimuli and events. While this information is vital to ensure proper functioning of the digestive tract, the enteric nervous system has no ability to produce conscious sensations. When Gershon's book, *The Second Brain,* came out, it sparked much speculation about the abilities of the enteric nervous system. Some even wondered if the second brain not only is capable of perception, but may also be the seat of our emotions and our unconscious mind. However, we can almost certainly say that these speculations were false. The sensory information from the gut is also sent to the brain in your head, and if you pay attention to these sensations you will be able to feel them.

Twenty-four hours a day, seven days a week, our GI tract, enteric nervous system, and brain are in constant communication. And this communication network may be more important for your overall health and well-being than you ever could have imagined.

Sensing with Your Gut

Take a bite of juicy hamburger, enjoy a piece of fresh, crispy baguette, savor a cup of New England clam chowder, or revel in the exquisite flavor of a good piece of chocolate. What do you taste?

The answer will be supplied to you by the collection of receptors located on the taste buds of your tongue. These molecules embedded in the outer membrane of a cell recognize the specific chemicals in anything you eat or drink, as a lock recognizes a key. When this receptor binds to such a chemical on a food item, it sends a message to your brain, and your brain constructs the particular taste from the streams of sensory information it receives from your mouth and tongue.

The taste receptors on your tongue can detect five distinct taste qualities, including sweet, bitter, savory, sour, and umami; the combination of these qualities in any bite of food determines its flavor. In addition, the texture of what you eat—the crunchiness of a carrot, the smoothness of yogurt, or the unique texture of a spaghetti squash—stimulates another set of receptors, which specialize in recognizing mechanical qualities of food. The combination of all of these sensations encoded in your mouth creates the experience that you know as taste. Food companies are masters in designing foods that maximize this experience.

Amazingly, recent research has shown that some of the same mechanisms and molecules that are involved in the taste experience are not limited to your mouth, but are also distributed throughout our gastrointestinal tract. Science has unequivocally shown that this is the case for the bitter and sweet taste receptors. In fact, evidence for some twenty-five different bitter taste receptors has been found in the human gut. While we know that the gut taste receptors have little or nothing to do with our taste experience, we also know very little about their functions in the gut-brain axis. However, these receptor molecules are located on sensory nerve endings and on the hormone-containing transducer cells in the gut wall (such as the serotonin-containing cells we discussed in the previous chapter), which puts them in a perfect location to participate in the gut-brain dialogue.

Some of these receptors are activated by specific molecules found in herbs and spices like garlic, hot chili pepper, mustard, and wasabi, while others respond to menthol, camphor, peppermint, cooling agents, and even cannabis. To date, twenty-eight of these so-called phytochemical receptors (receptors that recognize specific chemicals in plants) have been identified in the mouse intestine alone, and there is no reason to doubt that our human intestines have a similar or even greater diversity of receptors that are sensitive to a variety of chemicals contained in plants.

Most of us use spices and herbs to stimulate the taste receptors on our tongues, thereby enhancing the flavor of a meal. A growing number of individuals who believe in natural treatments consume herbs or their extracts specifically for medicinal purposes, and herbologists can tell you a litany of empirically derived health benefits for all of them. However, in many parts of the world, spices are an integral part of the culture: who could imagine Indian or Mexican foods without chili peppers, Persian food without an assortment of fresh herbs and yogurt, or Moroccan tea without peppermint?

It is plausible that regional and geographic differences in people's taste preferences for various herbs and spices have evolved to encourage their consumption, and provide protection against common illnesses prevalent in different parts of the world. For example, does the consumption of spicy foods in many parts of the developing world protect people from gastrointestinal infections? And does the consumption of fresh herbs in Persian dishes, or the obligatory consumption of peppermint tea after a meal in Morocco, prevent indigestion? Regardless of how we explain their prevalent use all over the world, these plant-derived substances link us and our gut-brain axis closely to the diversity of plants around us. The multitude of phytochemicals derived from a diet rich in diverse plants, combined with the array of perfectly matching sensory mechanisms in our gut, synchronizes our internal ecosystem (our gut microbiome) with the world around us.

Why are there so many sensors in our gut? Some receptors, like those that sense for sweet food, play an important role in the way we metabolize our food. When our sweet receptors sense glucose (created when carbohydrates are digested) or artificial sweeteners, they stimulate the absorption of glucose into the bloodstream, and the release of insulin from the pancreas. They also stimulate the release of several other hormones that signal to the brain and create a sense of satiety.

The function of the gut's bitter taste receptors remains something of a mystery. My colleague Catia Sternini, a neuroscientist at UCLA who's an expert on the enteric nervous system and who focuses on intestinal taste receptors, speculates that some of these receptors may respond to metabolites produced by intestinal microbiota, and that alterations in these receptors as a consequence of high fat intake and fat-related changes in gut microbiota could play a role in obesity. In a collaborative study, we have recently demonstrated support for this hypothesis in obese subjects.

There are other possible roles that have been proposed for the bitter taste receptors in the gastrointestinal tract. Their stimulation has been shown to result in the release of the gut hormone ghrelin, also known as the hunger hormone, which travels to the brain to stimulate appetite. I wouldn't be surprised if the ancient habit in many European countries of drinking a bitter aperitif before meals developed because of the aperitifs' ability to stimulate bitter taste receptors in the gut to release ghrelin and thus increase the appetite.

Think, too, of all the horrendous-tasting bitter herbal medicines employed in traditional Chinese medicine. It seems much more likely that their therapeutic effects have little to do with the bitter taste experience they give you, but are related in some way to the activation of one or more of the gut's twenty-five bitter receptors, thereby sending healing messages to your brain and body. Even more intriguing is the recent ev-idence that the same nasal olfactory receptors we use to enjoy the smell of roses, detect a carton of spoiled milk, or sniff out a good barbecue joint are also spread throughout the intestinal tract. Like the gut's taste receptors, these gut olfactory receptors are located primarily on endocrine cells, where they control the release of different hormones.

Since taste and olfactory receptors are located throughout the GI tract, rather than only in the mouth and nose, their original names—"taste" and "smell"—have become somewhat obsolete. Instead, scientists now understand that these recep-tors are part of a large family of chemical sensing mechanisms that are found in the lungs and other viscera, and play different roles depending on their location in different organs. Based on what we know today, I wouldn't be surprised if these chemical sensors are able to pick up messages from the different micro-bial communities living in these organs.

How does the nervous system obtain its share of this vital information from inside of your messy gut? It would hardly make sense for this high-performance data collection system to be immersed in the messy world of partially digested food and corrosive chemicals moving through the gut. In fact, it's not: the neurons themselves sit inside the gut lining, out of direct contact with the gut's contents, and rely on specialized gut-lining cells that do face the inside of the gut to sense events there. Those cells signal to intermediaries in the gut wall, in particular the various endocrine cells that in turn signal to nearby sensory neurons, in particular the vagus nerve. To date, a large number of different sensory neurons have been identi-fied that are each specialized for a specific aspect of gut sensa-tions and respond to a particular molecule released by the gut's endocrine cells. Each of these nerves will send signals to the enteric nervous system or to the brain.

The gut's endocrine cells are so abundant and so deft at signaling our nervous system that they play crucial roles in our health and well-being. Imagine for a moment that you could compress all these hormone-containing cells in your gut into one single clump of cells: it would be the biggest endocrine organ in our bodies. Endocrine cells that line the gut from the stomach all the way to the end of the large intestine can sense a wide range of chemicals contained in what we eat and which are produced by the microbiota. For example, when your stomach is empty, specialized cells in the stomach wall produce a hormone called ghrelin, which travels via your bloodstream or signals via the vagus nerve to your brain, where it triggers a strong urge to eat. On the other hand, when you're satiated and your small intestine is busy digesting your food, cells there release "satiety" hormones that tell your brain that you're full and it's time to call a halt to further eating.

In addition to the gut-brain communication channel involving the endocrine cells, there is another system involving our gut-based immune system and the inflammatory molecules these immune cells produce, the so called cytokines. The immune cells living in our gut are preferentially located in clusters in the small intestine known as Peyer's patches, and are also found in our appendix and scattered throughout the wall of the small and large intestine. The gut-based immune cells are separated by a tiny layer of cells from the space inside the gut, and some of them, the so-called dendritic cells, even extend through the gut layer, where they can interact with our gut microbes and with potential harmful pathogens. Most important, cytokines released from these cells can cross the gut lining, enter the systemic circulation, and ultimately reach the brain. Alternatively, the signaling molecules released from hormone-containing gut cells signal to the brain via the vagus nerve.

With so many mechanisms involved in informing our nervous system about aspects of the foods we ingest, it is becoming clear that our gut is designed to do far more than just absorb nutrients. The gut's elaborate sensory systems are the National Security Agency of the human body, gathering information from all areas of the digestive system, including the esophagus, stomach, and intestine, ignoring the great majority of signals, but triggering alarm when something looks suspicious or goes wrong. As it turns out, it's one of the most complex sensory organs of the body.

Total Gut Awareness

Whenever you consume food or drink, reports from your intestinal data collection system provide a variety of vital information to both the little brain in your gut (your enteric nervous system) and the brain in your head. Your big and little brains are both interested in obtaining these reports whenever you consume food or drink, but they're interested in different aspects of this information.

Your little brain needs vital information from the gut to generate optimal digestive responses and, when necessary, to eliminate toxins by expelling the intestinal content from either end of the GI tract by vomiting or diarrhea. These reports cover the size of the meal, the contents that are entering the gut (including chemical information such as fat, protein, and carbohydrate content, as well as concentrations, consistencies, and particle sizes). They also include intelligence revealing any signs of hostile intruders such as bacteria, viruses, or other toxins from contaminated food. When it obtains information about the high fat content of a rich dessert entering your stomach, it will slow the rate of gastric emptying and intestinal transit. When it obtains information about the low caloric density of a meal, it will speed up its emptying from the stomach to deliver enough calories for absorption. And when it obtains information about potentially harmful intruders, it will stimulate water secretion, change the direction of peristalsis to empty the stomach from its content, and accelerate the transit throughout the small and large intestine to expel the offending agent.

Your brain, on the other hand, is more concerned with your overall health and well-being and as such it monitors different cues from your gut and integrates them with a variety of signals from other parts of your body as well as information about your environment. It monitors what is going on in the enteric nervous system, but in addition is closely interested in your gut reactions, the state of the gut reflecting your emotions, the wrenching contractions of your stomach and colon when you are angry, and the absence of intestinal activity when you are depressed. In other words, the brain watches its own theater being played out on the stage of the gut. The brain almost certainly also receives information generated by the trillions of microbes living in the gut, an aspect of gut-brain signaling that only came into focus during the past few years. While the brain constantly monitors all sensory information coming from the gut, it delegates the day-to-day responsibilities to local agencies, in our case the enteric nervous system. The brain only gets directly involved in the action if an action is required by you, or if the situation poses a significant threat that warrants a brain response.

Through these various sensory mechanisms, your gut informs your brain every millisecond of the day, whether you're awake or asleep, about everything taking place deep inside you. It's not the only organ providing ongoing feedback to the central nervous system: Your brain continually receives sensory information from every cell and organ in your body. Your lungs and diaphragm transmit mechanical signals to the brain every time you inhale and exhale, your heart generates mechanical signals with each heartbeat, your artery walls send signals about blood pressure, and your muscles transmit information about their tone or tightness.

Scientists call these ongoing reports about the state of the body "interoceptive" information—information that the brain then uses to keep the body's systems balanced and functioning smoothly. Although interoceptive information comes from every single cell of the body, the messages the gut and its sensory mechanisms send to our brain are unique in their sheer number, variety, and complexity. Start with the fact your gut's sensory network is distributed over the gut's entire surface area, which is two hundred times larger than the surface area of your skin—about the size of a basketball court. Now imagine a basketball court with millions of tiny mechanical sensors that collect information about the movement of the players, their weight, their acceleration and deceleration, and about every jump and landing. Since the gut's signals also include chemical, nutritional, and other information, this metaphor only begins to describe the vast amount of information encoded as gut sensations.

The Information Highway for Gut-Brain Traffic

The vagus nerve plays a particularly important role in communicating gut sensations to the brain. The great majority of gut cells and receptors that encode gut sensations are closely linked to the brain via the vagus nerve. And much of the signaling of our gut microbiota to the brain relies on this pathway as well.

In the majority of rodent studies on the effects of gut microbial changes on emotional behaviors, the effects were no longer seen after the vagus nerve was cut. But the vagus nerve is more than a one-way communication channel: This nerve is a six-lane freeway, allowing rush hour traffic in both directions, though 90 percent of this traffic flows from gut to brain. The vagus nerve carries so much traffic because it's one of the most important regulators of our viscera, linking the brain not just to the GI tract but to all other organs as well.

The following patient anecdote illustrates how important this gut-brain communication system is for our overall well-being. During my training at UCLA, I met George Miller, who had long suffered from symptoms of a large ulcer in his duodenum—the first part of the small intestine. Not only was he miserable and in pain whenever his ulcer flared up, but he had to be hospitalized twice when his ulcer started to bleed acutely. After he had been suffering from these symptoms for years, the decision was made by his gastroenterologist to refer him to a surgeon to cut his vagus nerve, thereby removing its ability to stimulate acid production in the stomach. The personal stories and symptom histories experienced by patients like Miller following their vagotomies revealed a great deal about gut sensations and what happens to people when you deprive the brain of this vital source of interoceptive information.

In the early 1980s, the prevailing view in the medical and surgical community was that the simplest and most effective way to stop excess acid production and cure peptic ulcers was to cut the vagus nerve—a procedure known as a truncal vagotomy. These surgeries were done with little consideration for the massive flow of information through the vagus nerve from the gut to the brain, and the possible importance of this information flow to our overall well-being. Fortunately, surgeons rarely resort to such drastic procedures today, since we can now treat the great majority of ulcers medically.

In Miller's case, his surgery had been successful, in that his ulcer no longer troubled him. But the price he paid was enormous. From that point on, he suffered an array of unpleasant gut sensations. He felt full after even a small meal and endured constant nausea and vomiting, cramps, belly pain, and diarrhea, among other symptoms.

Miller's doctors could not explain his symptoms, which also included obscure symptoms such as heart palpitations, sweating, lightheadedness, and extreme fatigue, so they blamed his alleged neuroticism and labeled his constellation of symptoms a case of "albatross syndrome," a term once used to describe patients like Miller whose peptic ulcer surgery successfully treated their gastric ulcers but left them with a range of aversive gut sensation, lasting abdominal pain, nausea, vomiting, and poor food intake. But we now know that for many of these patients at least, their symptoms had a very solid physiological basis.

Today we know about the complexity of gut sensations and the crucial role the vagus nerve plays in transmitting these signals to brain regions like the hypothalamus and limbic brain regions, which in turn influence a wide range of vital functions such as pain, appetite, mood, and even cognitive function. In hindsight, it is easy to see that obstructing this vital information highway (like closing the 405 freeway in Los Angeles in both directions) would have profound effects on how someone feels when they wake up in the morning, or when they eat.

It's unlikely we'll ever know the exact mechanisms behind Miller's symptoms, since vagotomies are rarely performed today. On the other hand, there has been a renewed interest in studying the role of the vagus nerve in transmitting gut sensations to major control centers in the brain. Electrical or pharmacological vagal stimulation has been evaluated as a novel way to simulate gut sensations, and as therapy to treat a range of brain disorders, including depression, epilepsy, chronic pain, obesity, and even various chronic inflammatory diseases such as arthritis. These new findings further confirm the importance of vagal-gut-brain communication to people's health and well-being.

The Role of Serotonin

Among the most wrenching of gut sensations are those associated with food poisoning, and about forty years ago I became more closely acquainted with them than I had hoped. I was finishing a four-week backpacking trip in India. The journey had taken me past peaceful Buddhist monasteries and peach-tree-covered oases, and through deserted valleys and mountain passes from northern India to the foothills of the Himalayas. I had been subsisting on daily rations of lentil soup, rice, and butter tea, drinking water directly from pristine streams. I've rarely felt as elated as I did when I arrived in the hill station city of Manali, and to celebrate I departed from my usual routine and treated myself to a delicious and spicy meal at one of the local restaurants.

Early the next morning, I boarded the bus for a twenty-four-hour ride to New Delhi—a day that shall forever live in digestive infamy. Trying to control the gastrointestinal consequences of that meal was like telling an attacking pack of hyenas to lie down and roll over. The intensity of this experience engraved itself into the deepest layers of my emotional memory—a permanent reminder of just how powerful gut sensations (and their memories) can be.

Food poisoning occurs when you accidentally ingest a drink

or a meal contaminated with a pathogenic virus, bacterium, or a toxin produced by these microorganisms. Let's say it's the toxin of an invasive species of *E. coli*. In your intestine, the toxin binds to receptors located on the serotonin-containing cells. This signal immediately switches your GI tract's setting to "horrific vomiting and hurricane-like diarrhea." Some cancer chemotherapy drugs, including cisplatin, do the same thing.

This is an inbuilt survival mechanism: when your gut detects enough of a toxin or pathogen, your enteric nervous system issues an evacuation order to your entire GI tract aimed at expelling the toxin from both ends of your digestive tract—a smart reaction, if not a pretty one.

The reaction is driven by serotonin-containing cells in the upper gut, which are particularly important in the generation of gut sensations. When secreted under normal conditions, serotonin helps the digestive process proceed in regular fashion. It is released by subtle mechanical shearing forces exerted when the gut's contents slide along the GI tract and rub against what are known as enterochromaffin cells. Just like the other hormones contained in the endocrine cells of the gut, the released serotonin activates sensory nerve endings in the vagus nerve and the enteric nervous system (ENS), which in turn keep the ENS informed about what is moving down the intestinal tract, enabling it to trigger the all-important peristaltic reflex. A more concentrated serotonin release, such as occurs with food poisoning or in response to the chemotherapeutic agent cisplatin, on the other hand, will lead to vomiting, intensive bowel movements, or both.

My research group, working with a group from the Netherlands, found that in healthy subjects, a diet deficient in the amino acid tryptophan, essential for making serotonin, lowers brain serotonin levels, which increases activity of the brain's arousal network. These central nervous system changes are also associated with increased sensitivity to an experimental mechanical stimulation of the colon. The same serotonin-lowering diet had previously been shown to increase the likelihood of depression in at-risk individuals, including those with a family history of depression.

Serotonin is the ultimate gut-brain signaling molecule. Serotonin-containing cells are intricately connected to both our little brain in the gut and to our big brain. This gut-based serotonin-signaling system plays a key role in linking events in the gut related to food, intestinal microbes, and certain medications to the activity of our digestive system, and to the way we feel. On the other hand, the small amount of serotonin contained in nerves in the gut and in the brain plays crucial roles as well: serotonin-containing nerves in the gut play a key role in regulating the peristaltic reflex, while clusters of nerve cells in the brain send their signals to most regions of the brain, exerting an influence over a wide range of vital functions, including appetite, pain sensitivity, and mood.

Mike Gershon, pioneering researcher of the gut's serotonin system, likes to say that the only time you'll ever be aware of gut sensations related to the gut-serotonin system is when the news is bad—or in some cases very bad, like my hellish bus ride to New Delhi. But is that really so? Let's leave aside for a moment the dramatic events that unfold when a bacterial or viral infection triggers a massive serotonin release, or when an alteration in the gut's serotonin system produces IBS symptoms or diarrhea. Given the gut's enormous serotonin stores, located close to vagal nerve pathways that link directly to the brain's affective control centers, it's certainly conceivable that a constant stream of low-level, serotonin-related gut signals are being sent to our brain's emotional centers, in response to intestinal contents rubbing against the serotonin-packed cells, or in response to gut microbial metabolites. Even if these serotonin-encoded signals don't enter our conscious awareness, this low-level serotonin release could affect our background emotions and influence how we feel, exerting a positive "tone" on our mood—which in turn could explain why so many people experience a sense of contentment and well-being around the ingestion of an enjoyable meal.

Food as Information

All of this raises an important question: If the great majority of us don't consciously perceive the vast majority of our gut sensations—including the twofold distension of the stomach after eating a big meal, or the nutcracker-like contractions of the migrating motor complex when our gut is empty—then why does the gut need its specialized sensory apparatus?

The simple and scientifically supported answer is that these sensing mechanisms are essential to the smooth operation and coordination of basic gut functions such as gastric emptying, movement of food through the intestines, and the secretion of acid and digestive enzymes; to body functions related to food intake, such as appetite and satiation; and to our basic metabolism, including blood sugar control. These functional aspects of gut sensations most likely go back millions of years, to when tiny, primitive marine animals were "colonized" by microorganisms that helped them metabolize certain nutrients.

The other, more provocative answer to the question of why this gut sensory system exists has to do with the massive information flow from our gut to our brains—information that is not directly related to our gut functions and our metabolic needs, and that remains largely below our radar screens. The massive amount of gut-related information being sent to the brain, which includes a barrage of messages from the trillions of microbes living in our gut, gives the gut-brain axis a unique and unexpected role in modulating our health and well-being, our feelings, and even—as we'll see in Chapter 5—the decisions we make.

When we consider the scientific complexities of the various gut sensors and the vagus nerve, together with their functions in the digestive process, and place them into the overall context of gut sensations, a revolutionary picture of our eating habits emerges: not only is our digestive tract able to absorb most of the nutrients and calories contained in a meal (with our intestinal microbes taking care of the leftovers that our gut cannot digest), but the gut's sophisticated surveillance system can actually analyze food's nutritional content and, at the same time, extract the information needed for its optimal digestion. In other words, food comes with its own instructions for how to optimally digest it, and with a lot of fine print that until recently we didn't even know about, and are still trying to figure out the meaning of. This is true whether you are a vegan, pescatarian, omnivore, meat-meister, fast-food junkie, serial dieter, episodic faster—or even if you recently picked up a gut infection while traveling in Mexico. Most remarkably, the gut's intricate sensory system begins extracting this information the second the food enters our mouth—when taste receptors on our tongue and enteric nerves in our esophagus begin transmitting information about what we're ingesting—and continues doing so until the food ends up in our colon. And our gut does all this without interfering in any way with our daily functioning.

When we consider the dense distribution and vast area that the gut's sensory receptors occupy on the lining of our gut wall, it's clear that our gut is transmitting immense amounts of information to the brain at any given moment, both from the complex processes related to digestion and also from the input of 100 trillion chattering microbes in our intestinal tracts. In other words, when it comes to collecting, storing, analyzing, and responding to massive amounts of information, the gut-brain axis is a true supercomputer—a far cry from the plodding digestive steam engine it was once thought to be.

This realization is all part of our new, modern understanding of gut function, which includes a shift from a preoccupation with details of macro- and micronutrients, metabolism, and calories to the knowledge that our gut with its nervous system and its microbial residents is actually an amazing information-processing machine that greatly surpasses our brains in terms of the number of cells involved and rivals some of the brain's capabilities. Through our food supply this system connects us closely to the world around us, picking up vital information about how our food is grown, what we put into our soil, and what chemicals were added to it before we buy it in the supermarket. And as we will learn in greater detail in the following chapter, the gut microbes play a prominent role in this connection between what we eat, and how we feel.

MICROBE-SPEAK:
A KEY COMPONENT OF
THE GUT-BRAIN DIALOGUE

In the 1970s and 1980s, the leading research on gut-brain communication could be found at the Center for Ulcer Research and Education (CURE), on the campus of the U.S. Veterans Administration (now the U.S. Department of Veterans Affairs) in West Los Angeles. Founded by Morton I. Grossman, one of the preeminent physiologists of the digestive system, CURE was the mecca for scientists and clinical investigators worldwide who wanted to study stomach ulcers (which were a major health problem at the time) and, more generally, the fundamental mechanisms of how the digestive system operates. Books have been written and stories are still told about the center, its scientific breakthroughs, its founder and charismatic leader, and a disciple of Grossman named John Walsh.

When I arrived in Los Angeles in the early 1980s to work at CURE as a research fellow, my goal was to study the biology of communication within the gastrointestinal tract. The topic of gut-brain interactions had been completely absent from my medical school curriculum at Ludwig Maximilian University, in Munich, Germany. I had just completed my residency in internal medicine at the University of British Columbia, in Vancouver, and I couldn't wait to start what was initially conceived as a two-year research training fellowship to pursue my scientific interest.

At the time, John Walsh was a young, brilliant investigator who made a lot of his visionary decisions and discoveries based on his gut feelings—something I only realized much later in my life. He had a career-long interest in a group of then-mysterious signaling molecules called "gut hormones" or "gut peptides," which had first been isolated from the skin of exotic frogs and later from the guts and the brains of mammals. At the time, biologists thought that these signaling molecules worked as simple chemical switches that turned on or off the stomach's production of hydrochloric acid, or the pancreas's secretion of digestive hormones, or the gallbladder's ability to contract. But over the next few remarkable years in this cradle of modern gut-brain research, I would watch firsthand as our understanding of these signaling molecules evolved from simple on-off switches to a complex universal biological language that the trillions of microbes in our intestines use to communicate with our digestive system and even our brain.

A group of Italian biologists under the leadership of Vittorio Erspamer had discovered some of the first gut peptides in the skin of exotic frogs, where their role seemed to be to help deter predators. When an inexperienced young bird ingested such a frog, these molecules would be released in its GI tract, triggering a bad gut reaction that spoiled the meal and caused the bird to regurgitate the frog. This taught the young bird not to touch that type of frog in the future. And since the frog produced a peptide to which the bird's tissues reacted, the results proved that frogs and birds shared a chemical communication system.

Not long after the Italians reported their results, Viktor Mutt and his colleagues at the Karolinska Institute in Sweden searched for similar gut peptides in mammals. Eventually they extracted and purified these molecules on an industrial scale from cooked pig intestines, and they distributed them to interested investigators around the world. When these precious extracts were shipped in powder form to Walsh's laboratory, we treated them with awe, considering the amount of work and time that had been invested to isolate them. Later, we headed out to a Los Angeles-area slaughterhouse in the early morning hours, returning with containers of pig intestines from which we purified the gut peptides ourselves. When we injected one of these substances, a molecule called gastrin, we observed that the animal's stomach started ramping up its secretion of hydrochloric acid. Injecting another gut peptide—secretin—turned on secretion of digestive juices from the pancreas, while injecting the peptide somatostatin tended to turn both functions off. These gut peptides have also been called gut hormones, as they were able to reach distant targets in the body when injected into the bloodstream, just as hormones produced by the thyroid gland or the ovaries can send long-distance messages.

It didn't take long for scientists to discover that gut peptides were present not only in the intestine's hormone-containing cells, but also in the nerve cells of the enteric nervous system, which used them to fine-tune peristalsis, fluid absorption, and secretion. And when neuroscientists started looking in the brain, they found identical substances. There the peptides functioned as important chemical switches that could turn on and off various behaviors and motor programs involved in hunger, anger, fear, and anxiety.

The story took an unexpected turn in the early 1980s when

a group of scientists at the National Institutes of Health, led by visionary biologists Jesse Roth and Derek LeRoith, wanted to find out if microorganisms were capable of producing the same signaling molecules that Walsh, Mutt, and Erspamer had isolated from frogs, pigs, dogs, and other animals. They grew different microorganisms in a nutrient-containing broth, separated the microorganisms from the broth, and tested them for the presence of insulin, the hormone that signals our tissues to store energy from sugar after a meal.

In both the cells and the broth, they found molecules similar to human insulin—similar enough that the molecules stimulated lab-grown fat cells from rats to sock away energy from sugar. This dramatic result suggested for the first time that insulin did not originally appear in animals, as biologists had thought, but was already present in more primitive single-celled organisms that arose about a billion years ago.

I first learned about LeRoith and Roth's fascinating research when they sent extracts from other microbes to Walsh's laboratory at CURE, which used the radioimmunoassay tests to identify and quantify these molecules. These studies yielded surprising results: in addition to insulin, my colleagues found molecules similar to other mammalian gut peptides. Ancient microbial versions of many gut peptides and hormones, including noradrenaline, endorphins, and serotonin and their receptors, have since been identified.

Roth and LeRoith summarized their findings in a 1982 review article in the *New England Journal of Medicine*, writing that the signaling molecules that our endocrine system and brain use to communicate probably originated in microbes. Several years later, I became so intrigued by this evolving science that I decided to write a speculative review article myself, in collaboration with my friend Pierre Baldi, a brilliant mathematician then working at the California Institute of Technology. Even though a prominent linguistic professor at UCLA tried to convince me that you can only talk about language in the context of human communication, we gave it the title "Are Gut Peptides the Words of a Universal Biological Language." The article was published in the *American Journal of Physiology* in 1991.

When I showed the manuscript to Walsh, he jokingly said: "You're lucky this speculative paper was accepted for publication. These ideas are about thirty years ahead of their time." (As usual with his visionary statements, his prediction wasn't very far off.) In the article, we proposed that these signaling molecules represent the words of a universal biological language used not only by the gut, but also by the nervous system, including the little brain and the big brain, and by the immune system. Humans were not the only organisms using this cellular communication system: science had demonstrated that frogs, plants, and even microbes living inside our intestines used it as well. By applying a mathematical approach called information theory to the biological data, we even speculated about the amount of information that different types of signaling molecules—from hormones to neurotransmitters—were able to send between different cells and organs.

Unfortunately, the time was not yet ripe for the rest of the scientific world to realize the impact of these early discoveries. As Walsh predicted, it would take nearly three decades of research into brain-gut interactions for gut microbes to again take center stage.

The Downside of Early Gut Cleansing

Dahlia walked into my clinic in black clothing and dark sunglasses, as if she were on her way to a funeral. Having seen many such patients, I wasn't surprised by her appearance. The dark glasses may have been due to an extreme sensitivity to light, which is often associated with migraines. Or perhaps her outfit was a cloak that Dahlia, a forty-five-year-old woman, was wearing to try to hide her feelings of chagrin.

Dahlia had made the appointment to get help with her intractable constipation, but her medical problems were not limited to her bowel movements. Other symptoms included chronic pain all over her body, fatigue, and migraine headaches. During my conversations with her, it became clear that Dahlia was also chronically depressed, a situation that she attributed solely to her gastrointestinal issues. She told me that her difficulties with regular bowel movements dated back to infancy, when her mother gave her regular enemas—a common practice that many mothers of the era employed to ensure daily bowel movements in their children.

Regrettably, the only way Dahlia could guarantee regular bowel movements was by taking daily enemas and by receiving high colonics (a more extensive enema in which warm water is injected into the upper colon) on a weekly basis. Without the daily enemas, she said, she was unable to have any spontaneous bowel movements for up to several weeks at a time. Dahlia insisted that her colon was "dead" and was no longer able to transport any of its contents, and she was terrified that she would experience unbearable discomfort if she didn't induce a daily bowel movement. These facts, combined with her fear of discomfort from constipation, had fostered a strong belief that she would never be able to stop this enema regimen.

Dahlia had tried many previous therapeutic approaches, which had all failed, and treating her depression with various drugs only had a transient effect on her constipation. It seemed as if some unknown mechanism forced her gut-brain axis always back to its disturbed mode of communication. I ordered a series of diagnostic evaluations, none of which revealed anything that could explain her constipation. Most interesting was the fact that, based on a specialized test called a colonic transit study, the time it took for digestive waste to move through her colon was completely normal.

Dahlia was also convinced that her symptoms of anxiety, depression, fatigue, and chronic pain were caused by fermenting toxic waste products in her intestinal tract, and that her inability to rid herself of these waste products was having a major effect on her overall well-being. Many physicians upon encountering such a patient, with her constellation of symptoms and her bizarre-sounding stories, would perform a colonoscopy, and provide a prescription for the newest laxative and a referral to a psychiatrist. Today we know that such a strategy would ignore some important biological factors in the patient's symptoms. It is likely that the enemas Dahlia received as a young child interfered with the development of a normal gut microbial composition during her first years of life, resulting in long-lasting changes in the way her gut microbes communicated with her nervous system. Even though we still don't have the science to know exactly what these early gut microbial changes are that lead to symptoms like Dahlia's, her story strongly suggests that changes in the normal development of a healthy gut microbiome can put patients at risk of developing psychiatric symptoms as well as a lifelong miscommunication between the gut and the brain. I am convinced that in the future we will have therapeutic strategies to reverse such early programming errors of the gut-brain axis. Until then, a holistic treatment approach including a combination of pharmacologic and behavioral treatments to deal with her psychiatric symptoms, establishing a greater diversity of gut microbes through probiotic ingestion and a diet high in plant-based fiber, and the administration of herbal laxatives to stimulate fluid secretion in the colon is likely to be beneficial. Such an approach will also help to validate the patient's suffering and her unique story. In the case of Dahlia, this approach was able not only to gradually improve her gastrointestinal symptoms, but also to reduce her symptoms of anxiety and depression.

Over the years I've seen many patients with complex, seemingly unexplainable symptoms, and one of the important lessons I've learned is to listen to their stories in an unbiased way—no matter how odd they may sound, and no matter how poorly they fit into current scientific dogma. Medical students are not taught how to diagnose such patients, so it would be easy for even an experienced gastroenterologist to pass off Dahlia's misguided assumptions as a psychological aberration with specifics unique to her. But I suspect that in addition to the altered development of the gut microbiota-brain communication, her routine was in part a remnant of the ancient and all-too-enduring belief that toxic waste products accumulating in the colon play a role in all kinds of diseases and ailments, both physical and psychological, and that cleansing the colon is the essential remedy for this. This belief, called intestinal putrefaction or autointoxication, is nearly as old as papyrus, and its treatment was part of ancient healing traditions in every corner of the world.

Gut Suspicions

In ancient Egypt and Mesopotamia, people believed that rotting food in the intestines forms toxins, which then move through the body via the circulatory system and cause fevers, resulting in disease. To heal such ills, the Ebers Papyrus, an Egyptian medical text from the fourteenth century B.C., provides directions for using an enema to treat more than twenty different stomach and intestinal issues by "driving out excrements."

Ancient Egyptians claimed that the god Thot had taught them about autointoxication and about purifying the gut to avoid disease. This led the pharaoh to name an appointee known as "keeper of the rectum," whose job was to manage the royal enemas—one of history's first truly rough gigs.

Across the Red Sea in ancient Mesopotamia, Sumerians, members of the oldest known human civilization, also applied enemas to expel disease. So did ancient Babylonians and Assyrians, whose tablets from as early as 600 B.C. mention the use of enemas. Over in India, Susruta, the father of Indian surgery, was specific in his recommendations, describing in Sanskrit medical texts how to use syringes, bougies, and a rectal speculum. The tradition continued with Ayurvedic practitioners: the most important of the five detoxifying and cleansing Ayurvedic therapies was enemas to clear the lower GI tract. Ayurvedic healers also commonly used *niruha basti*, a type of medicated enema, to treat a variety of ailments, including arthritis, backache, constipation, irritable bowel syndrome, neurological disorders, and obesity. And in East Asia, Chinese and Korean healers were also concerned with the dangers of an unclean bowel. They prescribed enemas and colonic irrigation to manage the dangers of "internal dampness," which they believed could cause myriad problems, including high cholesterol, chronic fatigue syndrome, fibromyalgia, allergies, and cancer.

The founders of Western medicine had other ideas about how autointoxication affected the body, but they agreed that it was definitely not good. The classical Greek physician Hippocrates, for whom the Hippocratic Oath is named, documented using enemas to treat fevers and other bodily disorders. Hippocrates is also credited with the profound statement that all diseases start in the gut. Ancient Greeks adopted the Egyptian idea that rotting food inside us leads to disease-causing toxins, which brought about the idea of the four humors that had to be balanced to maintain health—an idea that held throughout the Middle Ages.

Why have humans been so obsessed for so long with the dangers lurking inside our guts? Many patients from different ethnic, educational, and socioeconomic backgrounds whom I see in my clinic strongly believe in this idea as well. They come convinced that some ill-defined and largely scientifically unsubstantiated processes in their GI tract are responsible for various digestive and other health problems. Over the years, such suspected processes have included candida yeast infections of the intestine, allergies and hypersensitivities to all kinds of dietary components, leakiness of the gut, and most recently, a perceived imbalance of their gut microbiota. Many of these individuals have embarked on often costly and cumbersome routines to combat these suspected ailments, including highly restrictive diets, supplements, and even antibiotics. The fact that they still come to my clinic with unabated digestive problems makes me wonder if any of the treatments they've tried have really done any good, or if they have at most simply relieved the patients' anxieties.

Humans have used all kinds of nonscientific explanations and rituals to reduce their fear and anxiety over health threats outside their control. Dietary cleansing rituals have been particularly popular, including juicing and special diets aimed to achieve a clean gut, a contradiction in itself. Today, these basic anxieties have been whipped up dramatically by the endless stream of stories from popular authors in popular publications—stories that make shifting claims about the ever-present dangers contained in what we eat. On the other hand, we now know from scientific studies that there is some validity to the fear of microbes in our gut and of the many substances they can produce. Just as there are criminals, scammers, and computer hackers in human society, there are microbes that don't play by the rules. Some of these transient microorganisms, in particular parasites and viruses, have their own agenda (usually procreation), and they ignore or even sabotage our health and wellness as they pursue it. They have learned to hack into our most sophisticated computer system, the brain, to use its emotional operating programs for their own selfish benefits.

To demonstrate how sophisticated these microbes can be, let me share a fascinating story that I first heard some fifteen years ago at a meeting of psychiatrists in San Francisco. There, Robert Sapolsky, a leading expert on the ill effects of chronic stress on our brain, gave an inspiring talk about an evil but clever microorganism named *Toxoplasma gondii*. In the talk, he described work published in 2000 by Manuel Berdoy and his research group at Oxford University. That study showed that *T. gondii* has its own agenda of survival and reproduction, which it pursues in a remarkably cunning and egotistical fashion.

While toxoplasma can reproduce in one place only—the gastrointestinal tract of infected cats—the parasite can actually infiltrate the brain of any mammal (including humans), by outsmarting the blood-brain barrier, which functions as a firewall to isolate and protect the brain from any unwanted influences. Once cats are infected, they then dispel this microorganism in their excrement. Thus gynecologists recommend that pregnant women keep cats and their litter boxes out of the house, and refrain from gardening in areas where cats may bury their feces in the ground. In toxoplasma's ideal world, cats excrete the parasite, and rodents subsequently ingest it. The parasite then forms round cysts throughout the rodent's body, and, in particular, in its brain. A cat in turn eats the infected rodent. The ingested cysts reproduce in the cat's gastrointestinal tract, the cat sheds newly hatched parasites in its feces, and the cycle of life continues.

Here is where the plot takes a fascinating turn, attesting to the remarkable cleverness of this microbe. Under normal circumstances, a pathogen from an infected rat would be very unlikely to wind up back in a cat because rodents instinctively avoid cats. But toxoplasma-infected rodents not only lose their instinctive fear of cats—they also begin to prefer areas that smell like cat urine.

To make this happen, the parasite's tiny cysts home into a specific region of the rat's brain with the accuracy of a cruise missile, and with minimal collateral damage. The target is the emotional operating system responsible for triggering the fear-and-flight response. This emotional and motor program normally causes the rats to flee at the first whiff of a nearby cat, but the parasite specifically eliminates rats' fear of cats. Infected rats continue to exhibit their normal defensive behaviors toward predators other than cats, and they perform normally on laboratory tests of memory, anxiety, fear, and social behavior. But when it comes to cats, the cysts don't stop there. They also boost activity in nearby brain circuits that control sexual attraction, causing toxoplasma-infected rats that smell cats to become sexually attracted to them. This clever hijacking of the rat brain's operating systems overwhelms the innate fear response by causing a sexual attraction to cat odor. In other words, the infected rats develop a fatal attraction to cats.

The evolutionary intelligence behind these strategies is remarkable. Pharmaceutical companies have spent billions of dollars to develop medications designed to perform the same tasks that toxoplasma accomplishes with such ease. Most of these investments have failed. For example, compounds developed to attenuate the fear response in anxiety disorders and to block the action of CRF, a molecule involved in the stress response, and compounds designed to boost libido in women with hypoactive sexual desire disorder have proven marginally effective, and they come with potentially serious side effects.

There are many other microbes that have developed astonishingly sophisticated ways of manipulating the host animal's behavior. When the rabies virus causes its host—such as a dog, fox, or bat—to become aggressive, it does so by infiltrating a specific brain circuit responsible for anger and aggression. This increases the chance of the infected animal attacking and biting another animal (or human), thereby transferring the virus contained in its saliva into the wounds of the victim. While the toxoplasma parasite and the rabies virus stand out in terms of the highly specialized knowledge of their host animals' nervous system, many other disease-causing microbes, including bacteria, protozoa, and viruses, have developed surprising and clever ways to manipulate the behavior of their host animals.

If a hacker had manipulated a company's computer system the way the toxoplasma parasite and the rabies virus manipulate the brain, we'd suspect that the infiltrator was a skilled hacker with in-depth knowledge of the system's code, and that he had perpetrated an inside job. Toxoplasma and rabies have evolved to understand the ins and outs of the mammalian brain-gut axis, and they have a detailed knowledge of mammalian emotional operating systems—and can manipulate them to achieve their goals.

However, parasites and viruses are not the only microbes with a remarkable ability to influence our brain. Over the last decade, researchers have found that some of the microbes living peacefully in our gut have equally impressive skills, though they don't use these skills against us. But still, their effects on the brain-gut axis are profound.

Do Microbes Mediate Gut-Brain Communication?

Just a few years ago, many of us studying brain-gut interactions thought we had identified all the essential components that contributed to bidirectional brain-gut-brain communication.

We knew about many of the ways the gut keeps tabs on digestion and on our environment: how it senses heat, cold, pain, stretch, acidity, nutrients in food, and other characteristics—so many, in fact, that our intestinal surface is arguably the largest and most sophisticated sensory system in our bodies. It seemed clear that those gut sensations were relayed to our little brain and big brain through the action of hormones, signaling molecules of immune cells, and sensory nerves, especially the vagus nerve. This new knowledge explained why our digestive system functions perfectly and without our awareness most of the time, why the gut reacts the way it does to a tainted meal, and why we feel good after a delicious meal.

We also knew that in managing digestion, the enteric nervous system—the little brain in your gut—acts as a local regulatory agency that stays in constant close contact with the federal authority, your brain, in case of emergencies. We had learned that when we experience emotions, specialized emotional operating programs in the brain create distinct dramatic plots that play out in our guts, causing a characteristic pattern of gut contractions, blood flow, and the secretion of vital digestive fluids for each emotion.

The clinicians among us were satisfied with our new knowledge that the disturbed communication between brain and gut plays a prominent role in functional gut disorders such as irritable bowel syndrome. And contrary to the view of the great majority of psychiatrists and most of my gastroenterol-ogy colleagues, I suspected early on that modifications in this communication system might even be involved in such nondi-gestive disorders as anxiety, depression, and autism.

Still, as happens often in science, our initial confidence turned out to be premature. Though we had uncovered much about bidirectional communications between the gut and the brain, it was becoming apparent that our bodies actually orga-nize gut reactions and gut feelings in the form of an elaborate brain-gut circuitry that includes the gut microbiota as an es-sential component. We had come to our earlier conclusions and made our predictions without taking into account this crucial role of the gut microbiota.

As it turns out, our emotionally triggered gut reactions do not remain tied up in the twists and spasms of our gut. They also trigger a myriad of gut sensations, which then travel back to our brain, where they can modulate or create gut feelings, and where they are stored as emotional memories of a par-ticular experience. And we have realized only in the last few years—to the surprise of scientists around the world—that our gut microbes play an integral role in this interaction between gut reactions and sensations.

As we now understand it, this mass of invisible life can communicate constantly with our brains through a variety of signals, including hormones, neurotransmitters, and myriad small compounds called metabolites. These metabolites are the result of the microbes' peculiar eating habits and are pro-duced when they feed on the indigestible leftovers of what we consume, on bile acids secreted by the liver into the gut, or on the mucus layer covering your intestine. In fact, in the con-versation between the gut and the brain, your gut microbiota engage in an extensive running dialogue, using a sophisticated biochemical language I'll call "microbe-speak."

Why do our gut microbes and our brains need such a so-phisticated communication system? How did microbe-speak develop? To answer these questions, I need to take you back in time—far back, to the earth's primeval, microbe-rich oceans.

The Dawn of Microbe-Speak

Approximately four billion years ago, life first appeared on earth in the form of single-celled microorganisms, the archaea. For the first three billion years of their existence, microbes were the sole living inhabitants of the planet. And there were trillions of them, more numerous than the stars in our galaxy. They floated in a silent but massive marine-based universe, packed with close to a billion different species of invisible microbes of different shapes, colors, and behaviors.

Over this vast stretch of time, through the trial and error of natural selection, these microbes gradually perfected the abil-ity to communicate with each other. To accomplish this, they manufactured signaling molecules to send signals, along with receptor molecules to serve as specific decoding mechanisms for these signals. In this way, signaling molecules released by one microbe could be decoded by another one nearby. And this signaling actually triggers a transient or persistent change in behavior in the receiving microbe. As Jesse Roth and Derek LeRoith discovered, many of these signaling molecules closely resemble the hormones and neurotransmitters that your gut uses today to communicate with your enteric nervous system and brain. Together you can think of these molecules as an an-cient and relatively simple language—just like the various bio-logical signaling dialects that different organ systems in your body use today.

About 500 million years ago, the first primitive multicellular marine animals began to evolve in the ocean, and some marine microbes took up residence inside their digestive systems. One of those tiny marine animals—the hydra—can still be found today in bodies of fresh water. This creature is little more than a floating digestive tract. It's a tube a few millimeters long, with a mouth at one end, a digestive system filled with microbes running down its length, and an adhesive disk at the other end to anchor the animal to a rock or underwater plant.

Gradually, the animals and microbes developed a symbiotic relationship, and the microbes found ways to transfer vital genetic information to their host animals. This information provided the host animals with a range of molecules that they were lacking, but which the microbes had learned to manufacture during billions of years of trial and error. Some of these molecules became the neurotransmitters, hormones, gut peptides, cytokines, and other types of signaling molecules our bodies use today.

Over millions of years, as primitive marine animals evolved into more complex creatures, they developed simple nervous systems in the form of nerve networks surrounding their primitive guts, not very different from the networks of the enteric nervous system that surround our guts today. The nerve networks in these creatures used some of the genetic instructions they received from the microbes to produce signaling chemicals, which allowed neurons to pass messages to each other and instruct muscle cells to contract. These were the precursors of our human neurotransmitters.

Amazingly, these simple nerve networks and their signaling molecules enabled the primitive animals of millions of years ago to respond to ingested food in a similar, programmed way as our guts do today. When they consumed food, they engaged in stereotypic movements equivalent to those of the human digestive tract: a series of reflexes that propelled ingested food from the esophagus through the stomach and upper intestine, and that helped to excrete unwanted intestinal contents. When these animals consumed toxins, they were able to expel them from either or both ends of their GI tract, the human equivalent of the vomiting and diarrhea associated with food poisoning. These early marine animals also contained cells that could secrete certain chemicals to help trigger their digestive reflex. These secretory cells may well be the ancestors of our enteroendocrine cells, the specialized cells in the gut that produce most of the body's serotonin and the gut hormones that make you feel hungry or full.

The new symbiosis between the tiny marine creatures and their resident microbes led to many benefits for both of them. The animals gained the ability to digest certain foods, obtain vitamins that they couldn't synthesize themselves, and evade or expel toxins and other dangers in their environment. The microbes in their digestive systems gained a contained, convenient environment in which they could thrive, and free transport from one location to another. That collection of microbes can be viewed as the earliest version of the gut microbiota in your intestines.

This symbiotic relationship between gut microbes and their hosts turned out to be so beneficial for both partners that it has been conserved in virtually every living multicellular animal on earth today, from ants, termites, and bees to cows, elephants, and humans. The fact that these basic digestive activities have persisted through hundreds of millions of years attests to the remarkable evolutionary intelligence that has been programmed into your gut and its enteric nervous system. It also makes it understandable why there is such an intricate relationship between our microbes, the gut, and the brain.

As more complex types of animals evolved, primitive nervous systems grew into a more elaborate network of nerves outside the digestive system. This network was separate from—yet still intimately connected with—the enteric nervous system, and it retained most of the signaling mechanisms. The elaborate new nerve network eventually developed into a central nervous system, which established its headquarters inside the cranium.

Gradually, central nervous systems took over management of behaviors related to the outside world that had originally been handled exclusively by the enteric nervous system, including the ability to approach or withdraw from other animals as circumstances warranted. These functions were eventually transferred to emotion-regulating regions of the brain, while the enteric nervous system itself was left in charge of the basic digestive functions, a division of labor that has persisted in our own gut-brain axis.

It's been hundreds of millions of years since a handful of microbes made initial contact with the primitive gut of a simple marine animal. But the long evolutionary journey that we've taken since then helps explain why today your own gut, including its enteric nervous system and its microbiome, continues to have such a powerful influence on your emotions and your overall well-being.

An Ancient Binding Contract

Take a moment now to ponder the wonders of your gut microbiota. This collection of some one thousand species of microbes comprises 1,000 times more cells than exist in your brain and spinal cord, and ten times more than the number of human cells in your entire body. Together, the gut microbiota weigh about as much as your liver, and more than your brain or your heart.

This has led some people to refer to the gut microbiota as a newly discovered organ, one that rivals the complexity of your brain.

The vast majority of gut microbes are not only harmless, but are in fact beneficial for our health and well-being; these are referred to by scientists as symbionts or commensals. The symbionts obtain nutrients from their hosts, and in exchange they help keep the gut in balance and defend against intruders. But there is a small number of potentially harmful microbes, called pathobionts, that reside in your gut as well. Under certain conditions, these untrustworthy microbes can turn their weapons against us. Pathobionts have molecular tools that serve as artillery for attacking your gut lining, causing inflammation of the lining or ulcers. This change of loyalty can be a consequence of changes in diet, antibiotic treatment, or severe stress, and it results in the abnormal accumulation or increased virulence of certain populations of bacteria, thereby transforming former symbionts into pathobionts.

Yet human gut microbes rarely resort to such aggressive tactics. Instead, they usually live in harmony with us, minding their own affairs, which include digestion, growth, and reproduction. Nor does our immune system turn its formidable weapons on gut microbiota. The simple reason is that the costs to both sides greatly outweigh the benefits. Instead, both sides provide services for the other. It's an ancient binding contract that functions as both a peace treaty and a trade agreement, ensuring substantial reciprocal benefits to all involved.

The symbiosis between the microbes and their hosts that developed in its simplest form millions of years ago continues in our bodies today. Microbes gain by being able to live a privileged life in our intestines, which comes with a constant supply of food, moderate temperatures, and unlimited free travel. They also gain a free connection to our internal Internet traffic—the constant flow of information transmitted by hormones, gut peptides, nerve impulses, and other chemical signals. This information allows them to keep track of our emotional states, our stress levels, whether we are asleep or awake, and which environmental conditions we are exposed to. Having access to this private information helps the microbes to adjust production of their metabolites not only to ensure optimal living conditions for themselves, but also to stay in harmony with our gut environment.

In exchange, the microbes provide us with essential vitamins, metabolize digestive compounds, called bile acids, that are produced by the liver, and detoxify foreign chemicals that our bodies have never experienced—so-called xenobiotics. Most important, they digest dietary fiber and complex sugar molecules that our digestive system can't break down or absorb on its own, and thus provide us with a substantial number of additional calories that we would otherwise lose in our stool. In prehistoric times, when people were more concerned with hunting and gathering enough food to eat than fitting into their skinny jeans, the extra calories that gut microbiota extracted from food helped them survive. But today, as we're awash in excess food and obesity is epidemic, the extra calories that gut microbes provide have become a liability.

Respecting the key points of this ancient binding contract has produced a remarkably peaceful and mutually beneficial coexistence between microbes and hosts that has persisted for millions of years. It is an astonishing accomplishment—we humans are light-years away from such a track record of harmony.

Microbe-Speak and Your Internal Internet

Your gut microbes are engaged in ongoing conversations with your GI tract, your immune system, your enteric nervous system, and your brain—and as with any cooperative relationship, healthy communication is essential. Recent research reveals that the disturbance of these conversations can lead to GI diseases, including inflammatory bowel disease and antibiotic-associated diarrhea, and obesity, with all its deleterious consequences, and may be involved in the development of many serious brain diseases, including depression, Alzheimer's disease, and autism.

The communication with the brain occurs in several parallel "channels" that use different modes of transmission. This includes molecules that can communicate with the brain as inflammatory signals, travel through the blood like hormones, or reach the brain in the form of nerve signals. Communication through these channels does not occur in isolation; as we will see, there is extensive cross talk between them. Your gut microbes can listen in on your brain's ongoing conversation and vice versa, and information flow through the biological channels that your gut microbes use to communicate with your brain is highly dynamic.

The amount of information that is allowed to travel through this system depends in large part on the thickness and integrity of the thin mucus layer lining the gut surface, the permeability of your gut wall (its leakiness), and the blood-brain barrier. Normally, these barriers are relatively tight, and the flow of information from gut microbes to the brain is restricted. But stress, inflammation, a high-fat diet, and certain food additives can make these natural barriers leakier.

To fully grasp what your microbes are doing inside you, for the moment consider the various microbial communication channels together as a conduit of information akin to the fiber optic line or cable that supplies your home with Internet service. The amount of information being transmitted through this conduit varies. At some moments, the microbes will be uploading relatively small "text documents," and the amount of transmitted information will be small; but at other moments, they'll be uploading a series of huge, information-dense video clips.

However, there are ways that this communication system works differently from your home broadband service. The service contract with your Internet provider caps the amount of information you can upload or download per second. In other words, you have a fixed bandwidth, depending on whether you signed up for the cheaper economy plan or the more expensive deluxe plan. The Internet connection between your gut microbes and your brain, in contrast, is highly dynamic, as if you had the economy plan for most of the time, but quickly switch to the deluxe plan when you are stressed—say, after you had dinner in a French restaurant that included an appetizer of foie gras and a filet of sole sautéed in lots of butter.

As we turn to the communication channels of microbe-speak, let's start by looking at the role of the immune system in the gut microbial signaling to the brain. There are several ways by which this microbe-immune system-brain dialogue can take place, and the consequences of altered interactions between the gut microbe and immune system have received a lot of attention recently, as disturbances in this complex dialogue have been implicated in many brain diseases.

One means of communication involves specialized immune cells known as dendritic cells, located just under the inner lining of the gut. Dendritic cells have "tentacles" that extend into the gut's interior, where they can communicate directly with the group of gut microbes that live near the gut wall. These immune cell sensors are a first line of detection. Under normal conditions, receptors on these cell parts—so-called pattern recognition or toll-like receptors (TLRs)—recognize various signals from benign microbes, assuring the immune system that all is well and that no defensive response is necessary. Our immune cells have learned to correctly interpret these peace signals from interactions with a large variety of gut microbes early in life. In contrast, when harmful or potentially dangerous bacteria are detected through these mechanisms, they trigger an innate immune response—a cascade of inflammatory reactions in the gut wall—to keep the pathogens in check.

Recent studies have shown that the mucus protecting the gut surface is produced by specialized cells in the gut wall and is organized into two layers: a thin, inner layer that firmly sticks to the cells of the gut wall and an outer, thicker, and non-attached layer. Together these two transparent layers are nearly invisible to the human eye, measuring only 150 microns across, or about one and a half times the thickness of a human hair. The inner mucus layer is dense and does not allow bacteria to penetrate, thus keeping the epithelial cell surface free from bacteria. In contrast, the outer layer is home to the majority of your gut microbes as well as complex sugar molecules called mucins, which serve as an important source of nutrients for the microbes, especially when you fast or you have less fiber in your diet.

When microbes penetrate the protective mucus layer that covers the lining of the gut, the molecules of their cell walls trigger the activation of immune cells beneath the gut lining, which then tailor the immune response depending on whether, or to what degree, the microbe poses a danger. One such molecule—lipopolysaccharide, or LPS—is of particular importance in this microbe-immune system dialogue. LPS, a component of the cell wall of certain microbes called gram-negative organisms, is able to increase the leakiness of the gut, thereby facilitating the transfer of microbes to the immune system.

In contrast to common belief, no gut infection with a nasty bacterium or virus is required to trigger such responses of the immune system. However, as scientists recently found out, several other mechanisms related to our diet and the resulting alterations in the composition of our gut microbia come into play. First, people eating a high animal fat diet have an increase in the relative abundance of such gram-negative bacteria in their gut, or Firmicutes and Proteobacteria, and are therefore more likely to chronically engage this immune activation mechanism. Secondly, a diet low in plant-based fiber reduces the abundance of a particular microorganism called *Akkermansia muciniphilia* inside of our gut. Under normal conditions, this organism plays an important role in regulating the quality and thickness of the mucus layer that is part of the barrier separating the inside of our gut from our immune system (the other part of the barrier is the intestinal wall itself). The bacterium does this by stimulating the mucus production by cells lining our intestines. The thinner the mucus layer, the closer the intestinal microbes get to the cells lining the gut, the leakier the gut becomes and the easier it is for the gut microbes to activate the gut's immune system. Thus when excessive dietary fat and greatly reduced dietary fiber intake—the hallmarks of the modern North American diet—has compromised the two natural intestinal barriers (the mucus layer and the gut lining) that keep us separated from the trillions of microorganisms in our gut lumen, the gut microbes or their signaling molecules can cross the gut lining in greater numbers, causing even greater engagement of the gut-based immune system, an inflammatory process that can spread throughout the body. This process has been referred to as metabolic toxemia.

No matter how the gut's immune system detects microbes, it responds by producing a number of molecules called cytokines. Under certain circumstances, these cytokines can cause local full-blown inflammation of the gut, as happens in inflammatory bowel disease or in acute gastroenteritis. But once the cytokines are generated in the gut, these signals can also be sent to the brain. For example, they can bind to receptors on sensory nerve terminals of the vagus nerve, the gut-brain information highway, and send long-distance messages into vital regions in the brain that can reduce your energy level, increase feelings of fatigue and pain sensitivity, and even make you feel depressed. And with milder degrees of vagal inflammation, the sensitivity of vagal nerve terminals to satiety signals decreases, compromising the normal mechanism that stops you from eating after a full meal. Interference with this mechanism is often a problem for patients with high dietary fat consumption.

Alternatively, cytokines may spill into the bloodstream, travel to the brain like a hormone, transverse the blood-brain barrier, and activate immune cells—called microglial cells—inside the brain. As the majority of cells in our brains are microglial cells, which respond to cytokines, this makes the brain a receptive target of gut-microbial-immune system signaling. Such long-distance immune signaling from the gut to the brain has been implicated in the development of neurodegenerative diseases such as Alzheimer's.

In addition to their elaborate ways of communicating with our immune system, microbes also use their metabolites to communicate with your brain in ways that are less dramatic, yet equally vital. Gut microbes are highly diverse and numerous—there are 360 microbial genes in the gut for every human gene—and can digest substances that we cannot. This produces several hundred thousand different metabolites, many that our digestive system doesn't produce itself. A large number of these microbial metabolites make it into the bloodstream, where they account for nearly 40 percent of all circulating molecules. Many are considered neuroactive, which means they can interact with our nervous system. The large intestine absorbs some of these metabolites, transferring them into the bloodstream, and more make it into the bloodstream if you have a leaky gut. Once in the circulation, the metabolites can then travel to many organs in your body, including the brain, as a hormone does.

Another important way microbial metabolites signal the brain is via the serotonin-packed enterochromaffin cells in your gut wall. These cells are studded with receptors that detect a variety of microbial metabolites, including bile-acid metabolites, and short-chain fatty acids, such as butyrate, that come from whole-grain cereal, asparagus, or your favorite vegetable dish. Some of these metabolites can increase the production of serotonin in enterochromaffin cells, making more of this molecule available for signaling to the brain via the vagus nerve. They can also alter your sleep, pain sensitivity, and overall well-being. In animal experiments, they were shown to influence the development of anxiety-like and social behaviors. And they may play a role in how good you feel after a healthy meal rich in fruits, whole grains, and vegetables, or how bad you feel after eating too many greasy potato chips or a basket of deep-fried chicken.

Millions of Conversations Within

What makes the role of the gut microbiota so intriguing and far-reaching is the fact that this mass of microbes is sitting right at the interface that separates our gut reactions and our gut sensations. Depending on the type of meal you just ate, or whether your gut is completely empty, the enteric nervous system alters the gut environment and manages digestion by controlling the acidity, fluidity, secretions of digestive fluids, and mechanical contractions of your GI tract. Thus gut microbes constantly adapt to regional shifts in acidity, secretion of vital digestive fluids, available nutrients, and how much time they have to digest them before they're excreted. Likewise, when stress or high anxiety causes the brain's emotional operating programs to create dramatic plots that play out in our guts, it alters gut contractions, rates of transit from the stomach to the large intestine, and blood flow. This can dramatically alter living conditions for microbes in the small and large intestine, and is probably one of the reasons why the composition of your gut microbes is altered during stress. In contrast, when you feel depressed and everything in your gut slows down, microbes sense these changes and activate genes that help them adapt to those shifting conditions.

Meanwhile, the digestive, immune, and nervous tissues are busy communicating with each other, using signaling molecules that include gut peptides, cytokines, and neurotransmitters. Crucially, all of these substances are elements of biochemical languages that, thanks to our long, shared evolutionary history, are actually distant dialects of "microbe-speak."

As we scientists got over our initial surprise at the pivotal role of gut microbes in brain-gut communication, and as we investigated this relationship further over the last few years, it became ever clearer that the brain, the gut, and the microbiome are all in constant, close communication. We began thinking of the brain, the gut, and the microbiome as parts of a single integrated system, with plenty of cross talk and feedback from one part to another. I refer to this system throughout the book as the brain-gut-microbiome axis.

For the entire twentieth century, scientists could not see our microbial partners because the great majority of them could not be grown in the laboratory. Until the advent of automated gene-sequencing techniques to identify classes of microbes and supercomputers to process the massive microbial data, we had no way of conducting extensive surveys to determine which microbes were there, which genes they collectively possessed, and which metabolites they produced. More specifically, we had only limited understanding of how the various players in the brain-gut-microbiome axis communicate with each other.

It's now clear that our gut microbes have more than just a privileged role in our body. As the prominent microbiome expert David Relman, of Stanford University, expressed it, "The human microbiota is a fundamental component of what it means to be human." In addition to their indispensable role in helping us digest large parts of our diet, it is becoming clear that gut microbes have an extensive and wholly unexpected influence on the appetite-control systems and emotional operating systems in our brain, on our behavior, and even on our minds. These invisible creatures in our digestive system have a word to say when it comes to how we feel, how we make our gut-based decisions, and how our brain develops and ages.

||||||||||||||||||||||||||||||||

PART 2

INTUITION

AND

GUT FEELINGS

CHAPTER

UNHEALTHY MEMORIES: THE EFFECTS OF EARLY LIFE EXPERIENCES ON THE GUT-BRAIN DIALOGUE

‖‖

It makes intuitive sense that growing up in a harmonious, protected family environment has a positive effect on a person's development. Parents all over the world strive to provide such an optimal setting for their children. But ever since the advent of psychoanalysis, we know that certain repressed, adverse childhood experiences can result in psychological problems later in life. Most of the time, such childhood experiences are out of the control of the parents. In her bestselling book *The Drama of the Gifted Child*, psychologist Alice Miller maintained nearly forty years ago that all instances of mental illness had their developmental origin in unresolved, subconscious childhood trauma, which could be physical or psychological in nature. Even though I was fascinated when reading Miller's book during my medical training in the early 1980s, it took me more than twenty years to realize that the connection between early adverse life events and adult health outcomes laid out in her book not only were relevant to the development of behavioral and psychological problems such as depression, anxiety, and addiction, but also might be relevant to the medical problems of my patients, in particular those with chronic gastrointestinal disorders.

Today, exploring a patient's first eighteen years has become an essential part of any medical history I take. And it turns out it is a very simple thing to do; it doesn't require a specialized psychoanalytical training, and it doesn't take much time. In many patients I often get more important clues about their illness from exploring early life experiences than from asking in great length about the details of their medical symptoms. I always ask my patients the simple question, "Do you think you had a happy childhood?" What is most remarkable is the fact that asking this question, and without any additional probing, I usually get an honest account of what traumatic experiences patients remember from their first eighteen years of life. Most of the time the patient had not made a connection between such experiences and their current medical problem. Also, as I have learned over the years, their answers reveal a lot about the origin and nature of the stomach problems they experience as adults.

More than half of my patients over the years have told me of family trouble while they were growing up. One of their parents may have been ill, or there was an acrimonious divorce followed by a prolonged custody dispute, or perhaps, in more extreme cases, a close family member suffered from alcoholism or drug addiction. Some confide in me that as a child they experienced verbal, physical, or sexual abuse from a parent or stranger.

Several years ago, a thirty-five-year-old woman named Jennifer came to see me. "I've been suffering from belly pain all my life, but it's gotten a lot worse this past year," she said. To better understand the nature of her abdominal pain, I asked about her bowel movements. She said some days she had to run to the restroom all the time, while at other times she'd be constipated and couldn't go for days. Her pain was worse on the days she had diarrhea, and her bowel movements would temporarily relieve it. As we talked, it became clear that Jennifer had been suffering emotionally as well. Since her early teens, she said, she had suffered from anxiety with accompanying panic attacks, and from recurrent bouts of depression.

Jennifer had seen several other specialists, including two gastroenterologists and a psychiatrist, and had undergone the usual battery of diagnostic tests, including endoscopies of the upper and lower digestive tract and a CT scan of her belly. None of the tests showed anything wrong. "The last two doctors I saw told me that there was nothing seriously wrong with me and implied that it was all in my head," she said.

Jennifer's doctors had prescribed the typical drug cocktail for such unexplainable brain-gut symptoms: the antidepressant Celexa and the acid-suppressing medication Prilosec. But they had also told her that she would have to learn to live with her symptoms, and that there was nothing more they could do for her. "I have almost completely lost my faith in the medical profession," she told me.

Doctors generally spend much more time asking patients about the details of their bowel habits and checking blood pressure and cholesterol levels than they do exploring their risk factors related to early life experiences. Yet a recent study of close to 54,000 randomly selected Americans showed that children or teenagers who experience adverse events have a higher like-lihood of suffering from poor health, a heart attack, stroke, asthma, and diabetes as adults. The risk for such negative adult health outcomes increased with the number of adverse experi-ences participants endured before the age eighteen. An earlier analysis of health records of a large health maintenance organi-zation, in the Adverse Childhood Experiences (ACE) Study, had reported similar findings, including a 4–12 fold increase in the risk for alcoholism, depression, and substance abuse and a 2–4 fold reduction in self-rated health. The questionnaire used in both studies, the ACE questionnaire, asked participants about traumatic events experienced in childhood—such as sexual, physical, and emotional abuse—as well as more general house-hold dysfunction related to the parents. The majority of these questions explored situations in which the stability in the fam-ily was disrupted and the nurturing interaction between the primary caregiver and child was compromised. Other studies have shown that the well-known association of poverty with poorer health outcomes is primarily linked to the health effects of the chronic stress that comes from living in a low socioeco-nomic status.

While the connection between a wide range of traumatic or unstable upbringings and negative health outcomes makes in-tuitive sense, it is only in the last thirty years that science has un-raveled the biological mechanisms that are responsible for this connection, opening up windows for reversing the detrimental effects of this early life programming. These scientific insights are not only stunning, but have far-reaching implications for our health. If more doctors were aware of these connections and took the time to ask their patients about their childhoods, they could uncover important risk factors and possibly even devise more effective integrative treatment plans to help them.

During my consultation with Jennifer, I asked her why she had been put on the antidepressant medication Celexa several years ago. We talked about her depression and anxiety. "It has nothing to do with my stomach pain," she insisted. I did not try to change her opinion on this sensitive subject, but I continued gently probing for factors that I suspected might underlie both her chronic digestive symptoms and her psychological symptoms.

"Do you think you had a happy childhood?" I asked her. Almost miraculously, the question unlocked a storybook of stressful tales. When Jennifer was still in the womb, her maternal grandmother was diagnosed with breast cancer, and the crisis distressed her pregnant mother. She witnessed her parents argue and fight for years when she was a girl, and they split in a bitter divorce when she was eight. Jennifer was not the only one in her family who had struggled with symptoms of depression and gut problems. Both her mother and grandmother had suffered from depression and anxiety on and off through their lives, and she remembers that they always complained about their "stomach issues." Jennifer's history tipped me off about the possible roots of both her brain and GI symptoms—and gave me confidence that I'd be able to help her.

Like many patients, Jennifer had never considered that her range of physical and emotional symptoms might be connected, that they might be tied to her stressful early life experiences, or that these experiences had programmed the interactions of her brain, the gut, and its microbes in a unhealthy way. But a growing body of science suggests that it's past time to integrate this idea into modern medical practice.

Programmed for Stress

In the spring of 2002, at a small scientific conference in Sedona, Arizona, two strong-minded physicians offered clashing views about the cause of stress-related disorders. I had co-organized the conference with Charles Nemeroff, a prominent psychiatrist then at Emory University, to explore the role of early life trauma in a range of chronic medical and psychiatric diseases. Sedona's secluded setting amid stunning red-rock wilderness helped lure leading researchers and practitioners from across North America.

On the second day of the conference, the well-known Canadian psychoanalyst and abdominal surgeon Ghislain Devroede took to the podium. Devroede specialized in treating patients who had suffered sexual abuse as children; he used psychoanalysis to surface their repressed pain and shame. Without such treatment, he maintained, the repressed emotion is buried in the body, causing physical symptoms. Then he told stories of patients with pelvic pain and intestinal disorders like chronic constipation he had treated, whose symptoms disappeared after they underwent psychoanalysis and faced their difficult pasts.

But Nemeroff, who had made his reputation studying the biological basis of major psychiatric disorders, was having none of it. He challenged Devroede. "We've learned that psychoanalysis is not very effective to treat the mental and physical consequences of early life trauma." The room grew tense. No amount of psychoanalysis would ever reverse the trace in patients' brains of early abuse, Nemeroff claimed. Most of the participants we'd invited agreed on this point. We no longer had to wonder about murky Freudian ideas about early sexuality or neuroses to help our patients heal.

Instead, science had shifted our thinking. We now have solid evidence that stressful experiences in early life, including a compromised interaction between the primary caregiver and his or her child, can leave lasting traces on his or her offspring's brain. We also know from extensive surveys in human populations that these changes can drive the development of stress-sensitive disorders such as depression and anxiety, and that they might also play a role in gastrointestinal pain syndromes like IBS. But questionnaire data and psychological theories are not sufficient to help affected individuals. In order to develop novel therapies aimed to reverse this early programming in patients, we needed to know how our earliest experiences alter specific neural circuits in our brains that underlie our response to a variety of stressful situations. This knowledge could only be gained from basic studies performed in animal models of early life adversity.

A breakthrough in our understanding began when psychiatry researchers in the 1980s realized that stress exerts the same biological effects on animals like rats, mice, and monkeys as it does in humans. A major focus of these animal studies was on the role of the interactions between the mother and her offspring, as such interactions were easier to model in the laboratory, compared to such uniquely human behaviors as verbal and emotional abuse, or marital discord.

For example, rodents, like people, have different temperaments: some are timid, others are social; some are intrepid explorers, others stick close to home. And some rat mothers—even genetically identical animals—are better than others at nurturing their offspring. A nurturing rat mom pampers her pups. She hovers over them with her back conspicuously arched and legs splayed outward, allowing them to switch nipples, and she spends a lot of time licking and grooming them. A more negligent rat mom lazes on her side or lies on top of her pups as they struggle to nurse. This keeps them from switching nipples or wiggling, both of which are good for infant rats.

In landmark experiments that began in the late 1980s, Michael Meaney, a neuroscientist at McGill University, in Montreal, studied how the interactions between rat moms and pups played out in the lives of the pups. His research team took genetically identical rat mothers and videotaped and analyzed their behaviors while the pups were infants. Then they let the pups grow up, and checked how the pups of nurturing rat moms fared compared with the offspring of stressed-out moms.

The pampered pups grew into adults that were more laid-back, less reactive to stress, and less prone to addictive behaviors, such as overdoing it when given a free supply of alcohol or cocaine. They were also more social with other rats, more daring, and more willing to explore new places. Pups of stressed, negligent moms grew into loners prone to the rat equivalents of anxiety, depression, and addictive behaviors. Studies of monkey moms and their infants turned up similar results. Stressed macaque infants whose moms are inconsistent, erratic, and sometimes dismissive grow up timid, submissive, fearful, less gregarious, and more prone to depression than their better-nurtured peers. These early findings were the beginning of a paradigm shift in our understanding of how experiences in childhood can affect our health and the dialogue between the gut and the brain.

In another animal study, neuroscientists Paul Plotsky from Emory University and Michael Meaney studied rat pups whose moms were either naturally nurturing or naturally negligent. After the pups grew up, they stressed them by restraining them for a few minutes in tiny, formfitting stalls. The better-nurtured rats had lower levels of corticosterone, the rat stress hormone. (Cortisol is the human equivalent.) They also had hormonal changes in their blood and brain that keep the body's stress response from running wild. It turned out that pups that had been licked and cuddled released several hormones, including growth hormone, that are essential for the young brain's development.

In the meantime, a large body of scientific evidence has accumulated that confirms the close relationship between a mother's stress level and the way the nervous system of the child will react to stress later in life. In various laboratory situations that have been designed to stress an animal mother—and thus affect her nurturing behavior toward her young—researchers have found that the stress-induced changes in the mother's behavior programs the offspring's brains to become more responsive to stressful situations, and create more anxiety in adults. No matter what the initial stressor is or what kind of animal is involved, the effect is similar. The more severe the stress on the mother, the worse her behavior toward her young, turning even once-nurturing moms into negligent mothers. Stressed moms trampled their pups, didn't give them enough time to nurse, and licked and cuddled them less. Some were so stressed out that they killed their pups and ate them!

What was even more remarkable than observing the consistent negative effects of maternal stress on their young's behavior were the insights into the biological mechanisms underlying these behavioral changes. Studying the brains of affected mice has revealed dramatic structural and molecular changes. Whole brain circuits and connections developed differently depending on the mother's behavior, and several neurotransmitter systems involved in these connections were altered. The neglected animals had greater production of the stress molecule CRF, and less efficient systems that can regulate the stress response, including the signaling circuit involving the neurotransmitter GABA (gamma-aminobutyric acid) and its receptors. Because of these changes, even an antianxiety drug as strong as Valium did little to ease their stress.

Largely as a consequence of my daily interaction with patients who report experiencing adverse early life events—studies suggest that such a history is reported by up to 40 percent of healthy people and up to 60 percent of IBS patients—my research during the past twenty years has focused on better understanding the link between altered brain-gut interactions and early life adversity.

Early Stress and the Hypersensitive Gut

Not long after publication of the first studies of how mothering can program the brains of young rats, I received an invitation to a conference organized by the American College of Neuropsychopharmacology that brings together biological psychiatrists from across North America. Honored by the invitation, I participated in a mini-symposium on stress mechanisms, where I met Paul Plotsky, the neuroscientist from Emory University, for the first time. Listening to his presentation about his work on stress in mother rats and how it alters the biology and behavior of their young, I immediately wondered how his findings could be applied and, more important, offer some benefit to my patients with chronic gastrointestinal disorders.

Shortly after the conference I flew to Atlanta to explore possible ways we could collaborate. It was a rainy, hot Atlanta evening, and over dinner at a restaurant and a drink at his house, Paul and I talked for hours about what his work meant not only for stress-related gut disorders, but also for mind-body science in general. I mentioned my patients' gut disorders, pain, and other psychological symptoms. "That's me. I have all of that," he joked. I wondered aloud whether my patients' symptoms could be caused by childhood programming of their brain-gut axis. And I decided to spend some time in Paul's lab to explore this theory.

When I planned these experiments, I had IBS patients like Jennifer in mind. We knew by then that adverse childhood events predisposed adults to anxiety, panic attacks, and depression. But other than a few reports linking IBS symptoms to past sexual abuse, no one knew whether these sorts of events caused gastrointestinal pain and altered bowel habits, and we had absolutely no idea if alterations in our gut microbes were involved in these processes.

When we stressed mother rats by separating them from their pups for three hours a day during the first weeks of life, as Plotsky had, the pups later showed many IBS-like features. In IBS patients, normal gut activity can cause abdominal pain, cramping, and visible bloating of the stomach—all of which stem largely from a hypersensitive and hyperresponsive gut. The majority of patients also have elevated levels of anxiety, and a good percentage suffer from an anxiety disorder or depression. In our experiments, the rats that had experienced a less nurturing childhood presented with similar traits. The animals were more anxious, their intestines were more sensitive, and when stressed they would excrete more small stool pellets, the rat equivalent of diarrhea. Anyone who's ever had to run to the bathroom before a big presentation or job interview knows the feeling, but IBS patients—and our rats—suffer from such stress-induced symptoms all the time.

Remarkably, a chemical that blocks the action of the chemical CRF, the master switch in the brain that we know is increased by early life stress, banished all their symptoms: their stress-related behaviors, gut hypersensitivity, and stress-induced diarrhea. Unfortunately, even though such drugs could one day treat IBS and many other stress-sensitive disorders, efforts to develop safe and effective medications targeted at the CRF signaling system in the brain-gut axis have been unsuccessful so far. Many scientists involved in this effort, including those in my own laboratory, have struggled to understand this failure. Is the story in humans more complicated than originally thought? While basic scientists are always quick to make immediate conclusions about possible novel drug treatments based on their rodent experiments, our brains are not only much larger than those of rodents, but they have circuits and regions that are either underdeveloped or don't even exist in the brain of a mouse, such as our prefrontal cortex or the anterior insula. So I decided early on that if we wanted to determine the relevance of the groundbreaking observations made in animals for a better understanding of medical symptoms in humans, it was essential to look directly at the brain of human subjects who had experienced early adversity.

With this goal in mind, we used the power of neuroimaging to look directly into the brain of living human subjects. Using this technology, we imaged the brains of one hundred healthy adults who before turning eighteen had experienced neglect; verbal, emotional, or physical abuse; serious parental illness or death of a parent; or divorce of their parents or other serious family strife. I was amazed to discover that even in healthy individuals who exhibited no symptoms of anxiety, depression, or gut dysfunction, their brain scans showed altered brain structures and altered neural activity in brain networks that enable us to appraise the danger of a situation or the meaning of a particular body sensation. This so-called salience system also plays an important role in predicting positive or negative outcomes of situations, and is an integral part of our gut-feeling-based decision making. These findings were remarkable in several respects. We had demonstrated for the first time in humans that our brains become rewired in response to adverse experiences early in life—and that rewiring can persist throughout our lifetime. As we saw these changes in completely healthy people, we also learned that such changes are not necessarily accompanied by a particular health problem. While such individuals are more likely to worry, to be anxious, and to be more risk-averse, they may never encounter the GI problems that Jennifer suffered from. Could it be that these altered brain networks simply put us at a higher risk of developing a wide range of stress-sensitive disorders, including IBS? Our studies have shown that IBS patients have brain network alterations that play an important role in their hyperresponsiveness to psychological stress, and to normal signals coming from the gastrointestinal tract in response to a meal.

How Stress Effects Can Be Transmitted from One Generation to the Next

One of the speakers at our Sedona conference was Rachel Yehuda, a prominent neuroscientist at New York's Icahn School of Medicine at Mount Sinai. She talked about her groundbreaking findings that adult offspring of Holocaust survivors who had grown up without the experience of trauma themselves had a greater risk of developing psychiatric disorders such as depression, anxiety, and post-traumatic stress syndrome. Since then, several additional studies have shown similar types of "intergenerational transmission" of stress and adversity, including studies of the offspring of individuals who had to evacuate the World Trade Center on 9/11, or who had suffered through the Dutch famine during World War II. How could children raised in a safe and supportive environment by parents who had experienced the unspeakable trauma be more at risk for developing behavioral changes that are normally only seen in individuals who experience such trauma themselves?

In Meaney's rat studies, when the daughters of stressed, neglectful rat moms became mothers themselves, they behaved no better toward their own pups. His study found that the effect could last for several generations, suggesting that the stress experienced by the mother, and the ensuing effect on her behavior toward her pups, could somehow be passed to their offspring.

The question was how. It took several years of careful laboratory detective work by Meaney and molecular biologist Moshe Szyf of McGill University to unravel the mystery, but the results revolutionized biology. They found that very specific aspects of rat mother-pup interactions (such as the arched-back nursing or licking) can chemically modify a newborn's genes. Inside the cells of neglected rat pups, enzymes attached chemical tags called methyl groups to their DNA. This mode of inheritance is called epigenetic, since the tags sit on the DNA, and the prefix *epi-*, from ancient Greek, means "upon." It differs from the conventional, genetic mode of heredity because the tagged gene still carries the same information, and makes the same protein. But when it's tagged, it has a hard time doing so.

Here's another way to look at the underlying biology: If the human genome—the collection of all of our genes—is the book of life, then a brain cell, liver cell, and a heart cell each reads different sections of the book. Epigenetic tags are the bookmarks and highlighting that tell a brain cell to read one passage of the book and a liver or heart cell to read another.

Poor mothering altered just a few of the bookmarks and highlights. But some of the tagged genes altered brain signaling, which made the adult daughters poor mothers themselves. This caused their own pups to tag their genes, and the cycle continued. We now know that this epigenetic editing of our genes can affect not only cells and mechanisms that determine how our brain develops, but also our germ cells or gametes, which carry the genetic information passed on to our children. The discovery of epigenetics ended a long-running debate over the degree to which nature or nurture causes stress-related diseases. Epigenetics violated everything modern biologists had believed about inheritance.

Remember that Jennifer's mother and grandmother had suffered from symptoms very similar to her own: depression, anxiety, and belly pain. Most physicians would take this as evidence that genes for these disorders "ran" in Jennifer's family. But a study performed of nearly twelve thousand twin pairs by Rona Levy at the University of Seattle, Washington, to determine the role of heredity in IBS symptoms questioned such a simple explanation. Not surprisingly, in genetically identical twins there was a higher likelihood that both twins suffered from IBS symptoms, compared to such concordance in dizygotic twins. This finding confirmed that genes play an important role in the development of IBS. However, Levy also found that having parents with a diagnosis with IBS was a stronger predictor of an IBS diagnosis in their children than having a twin with IBS. This means that mechanisms *other than genes* play a crucial role in the intergenerational transmission of clinical diagnosis. While other interpretations are possible (for example, the role of social learning), it is plausible that epigenetic mechanisms also play an important role in explaining the common family history of stress-sensitive disorders such as IBS.

Epigenetics not only called into question the prevailing dogma that an acquired trait could not be transmitted genetically; it also overturned dogma in psychiatry. For a century, psychiatrists believed that the unconscious mind contains buried feelings about early trauma, hidden desires, and unresolved dynamics between mother and child. These unresolved issues could cause psychological problems in adults, according to psychoanalytic theory, as well as stress-related diseases like IBS in patients like Jennifer.

We know now that many of these Freudian ideas are flawed.

Science solidly supports the view that adversity experienced early in life, including poor mothering, can hardwire heightened stress sensitivity in our brains, and that this programming can be transmitted over generations, perpetuating a vulnerability for a variety of brain disorders.

DOES YOUR CHILD HAVE A STRESSED BRAIN-GUT AXIS?

If your grade school daughter is anxious, if your teenage son gets so stressed out over quizzes and finals that he smokes pot to calm himself, only to take stimulants to overcome his ADHD symptoms, or if your child suffers from IBS symptoms, is it because you failed to sufficiently nurture them when they were young? Rest assured, the answer to these questions is a definite NO. Women nurture their newborns through breastfeeding, touch, and other forms of body contact, behaviors akin to the arched-back nursing, licking, and grooming that nurture healthy brain development in young rats.

However, human brains are immensely more complex than rat brains. And there are many examples of highly successful and happy individuals, who had stressed-out single moms struggling to make a living, or who have overcome even the most severe forms of early adversity. In humans, there are many factors that can protect us from the negative effects of early life stress, ranging from genetic factors, to buffering effects during early development. Stay-at-home dads, grandparents, older siblings, nurturing nannies can all help create a supportive, stable family environment, helping children overcome the effects of early adversity. And keep in mind that the time window during which the development of the stress system is impacted by outside influences lasts up to twenty years in humans.

And even if such buffering factors are not present, as humans we have many tools at our disposal that allow us to partially reverse the programming from early stress and trauma in ways that rats and other animals cannot. For example, several mind-based therapies, including cognitive behavioral therapy, hypnosis, and meditation, have all been shown to change the way we appraise situations and body sensations. All of these therapeutic modalities are not just psychological treatments; they also have the ability to improve the cortical control over emotional and stress-generating circuits in our brains. We now know that such therapies can alter the structure and function of the brain's networks involved in attention, emotional arousal, and salience assessment, primarily by strengthening our brain's prefrontal cortex.

The Gut Microbiome Under Stress

Up to now, much of our discussion has focused on the programming of our brain circuits by early life experiences. There is no question that in vulnerable individuals, a disturbance of a stable, nurturing environment during the first two decades of life can change the development of the adult brain and behavior. These changes can be understood as an early programming of our nervous system in a way that reflects our first negative interactions with the world. And we shouldn't forget that a hyperreactive stress system may provide some advantage if one is born into a dangerous environment. But what benefit is there to suffer from IBS symptoms throughout life as a "side effect" unintended by evolution? And what are the consequences of such a programmed brain-gut axis for our interactions with the trillions of microbes living in our gut?

We have made tremendous progress in understanding the relationship between early adversity, changes in the cross talk between the gut and the brain, and the role of the gut microbiome in these interactions. It is becoming clear that early life stress not only affects the brain and the gut, but also has a profound effect on the gut microbiome as well.

Studies have shown that when adolescent rhesus monkeys leave their mothers for the first time, they develop separation anxiety and diarrhea—just like many teenagers do when they leave home for college. Diarrhea develops because stress causes the gut to contract more forcefully and propel ingested food faster throughout its length. In addition, stress increases the secretion of various digestive juices into the gut. These stress-induced changes in gut function have dramatic effects on the living conditions for gut microbes. In response, fecal bacteria numbers drop significantly, and the ranks of lactobacilli, a genus of protective bacteria, thin the most. Pathogenic microbes such as Shigella or E. coli are emboldened, opening the door to gut infections. The stress hormone norepinephrine also makes such invaders more aggressive and more persistent. In the monkey experiments, though, the stress effects were temporary. By the end of the first week, when the young monkeys adapted to their newfound independence, their gut lactobacilli levels returned to normal levels. Since the effect on the gut microbiota was transient, does it matter? Do these transient microbial changes have any effect on our brains?

In a recent study by Premysl Bercik's group at McMaster University, in Hamilton, Ontario, the investigators confirmed our earlier findings in the same animal model that poor mothering was responsible for the increased responsiveness of the gut to stress, consistent with alterations in the brain's stress circuits. But remember that animals with compromised maternal care also showed other changes, such as anxiety and depression-like behaviors. Bercik's group identified for the first time the special role of the gut microbiota in the development of these behavioral changes. It was only these "psychological" consequences of compromised maternal behavior that were dependent on the alterations in the gut microbiota and their metabolites, whereas the changes in gut reactivity were related to the increased stress responsiveness in animals. If these remarkable findings can be confirmed in human studies, it would have profound implications not only for our full understanding of the role of the gut microbiota in stress-related psychiatric disorders, but also for the treatment of patients like Jennifer and others with stress-sensitive disorders and a history of early adversity. Modulating the gut microbiota with dietary interventions and with pre- and probiotics, thereby reversing some of the effects of the altered gut microbes on the brain, could become an important tool in the integrative treatment plan.

Stress in the Womb

It has long been known that if you're pregnant, your stress level can jeopardize your baby's future health. Babies born to highly stressed mothers develop more slowly, weigh less at birth, and are more vulnerable to infections. However, until very recently little has been known about the potentially detrimental effects of maternal stress on the behavior and brain development of the offspring.

Two lines of evidence pinned some of these stress effects to changes in our microbial companions. First, monkey experiments showed that maternal stress alters our gut microbiota.

Neurobiologist Chris Coe, of the University of Wisconsin-Madison, exposed pregnant rhesus monkeys to alarming noises on and off for ten minutes every weekday for six weeks. This stressed the monkey moms about as much as traffic, noise, or working until a few days before delivery stresses a pregnant mom in a big city. Surprisingly, newborns of the stressed-out monkey moms had much fewer good gut bacteria—lactobacilli and bifidobacteria—than newborns of monkey moms who'd been left in peace.

At first it was unclear how maternal stress could alter the newborn's gut microbiota, since the unborn baby's gut is largely devoid of microbes. But now we know that stress can alter the mother's vaginal microbiota, which in turn has a major influence on the newborn's gut microbes. Neuroscientist Tracy Bale, of the University of Pennsylvania, and her team stressed out pregnant mice by exposing them to a series of uncomfortable situations, including the lingering odor of a fox. Bale's laboratory had previously shown that the same prenatal stress paradigm resulted in major neurodevelopmental changes in male pups in emotion- and stress-regulating brain networks.

In addition to what we already know about the effects of stress on an animal's *gut* microbiota, the investigators found major changes in the *vaginal* microbiome of the stressed moms, in particular a reduction in lactobacilli. It had long been known that stress-induced reductions in vaginal lactobacilli can change the acidity of the vaginal environment and predispose women to vaginal infections. But why on earth would these stress effects on the vaginal microbiome be so important for the young animal's brain development and behavior?

Because the mother's vaginal microbes first seed the baby's gut microbiota, these mice gave birth to babies with fewer lactobacilli in their guts, just as the stressed monkey moms had babies with reduced lactobacilli in their intestines. This stress effect is particularly concerning as it occurs at a crucial time, when the complex architectures of both the baby's gut microbiome and its brain circuits are being programmed for a lifetime.

But the mouse mom's stress didn't just affect her pups' gut microbes—it affected their brains as well! Bale's team analyzed the mix of molecules produced by the baby mice's microbiota. They found changes in molecules that supply the animals with energy, which the infant's brain consumes voraciously, and a short supply of amino acids, which help the fast-developing brain grow and form new connections between certain brain regions.

What are the implications of these laboratory studies for women experiencing pregnancy and motherhood today? Many adult brain disorders, including anxiety, depression, schizophrenia, autism, and most likely IBS, are now considered neurodevelopmental disorders, meaning that the basic brain changes start very early in life, many of them already in utero. As we have learned, stress is a major factor that influences these neurodevelopment changes, and there are at least two major pathways by which early adversity can affect the brain-gut axis: one is by epigenetic modification of the stress response system and the brain-gut axis; the other one is through stress-induced changes in the gut microbiota and their products, which can further affect the brain. This means if we really want to have a major and long-lasting impact on the development and trajectory of these devastating diseases, interventions will have to start very early in life. Once the adult patient comes to the clinic with the full-blown syndrome, most treatments will be largely symptomatic and transient, while it is more challenging to get long-lasting therapeutic success. But as we will see in the case of Jennifer, the new understanding made possible by recent science opens up more effective treatment options for the adult patient as well.

Microbes for a Healthy Start

Years before I began my research career, I witnessed an astounding event that even today sways my thinking about our microbial companions. On a winter break from college, I had been lucky enough to join a documentary filmmaker on an expedition to film the Yanomami people, who live on the upper Orinoco River, deep in the rain forest of Brazil and Venezuela. One moonlit night, I lay in my hammock near my host Yanomami family, listening to the sounds of the jungle and unable to sleep. I stood up, heard a noise nearby, and walked a few steps into the surrounding forest. There I saw a fifteen-year-old native woman alone, squatting over a large banana leaf on the ground, giving birth to her child in nearly complete silence. After delivering the baby, she severed the umbilical cord with a sharp object.

Here was a child being born naturally, without any help or medical intervention, and so quietly that no one else in the entire village seemed to notice. The circumstances of this childbirth were a world away from our modern hospital deliveries, which I had experienced during my medical training: no sterile hospital environment, no ob-gyns to treat the mother's vagina with antiseptics to "cleanse" it of microbes. Instead the newest Yanomami had been exposed not only to the mother's vaginal microbiome but also to all the microbes on her (unwashed and unsanitized) hands, on the banana leaf and in the soil. Yet over the next weeks, the baby cuddled by both parents seemed perfectly healthy.

In the Western world, childbirth goes a lot differently, of course, and the roots of our own practices run deep. At the turn of the twentieth century, French pediatrician Henry Tissier proposed that human infants develop within a sterile environment, and that our first contact with microorganisms occurs when we are exposed to the vaginal microbiota during birth. This view has remained dogma for more than one hundred years, but today there's good reason to doubt it.

Even in healthy pregnancies, maternal gut bacteria—most of them beneficial—have turned up in umbilical cord blood, amniotic fluid, meconium, and on the placenta, according to recent work. As the time of delivery nears, the vaginal microbiota changes a great deal. The diversity of microbial species decreases, and a lactobacillus species normally found in the small intestine becomes more prevalent. During birth, a baby born naturally is exposed to the mother's vaginal microbiota, including this lactobacillus species, providing the key source of microbes to colonize the infant's gut. In this way, your mother's distinct set of vaginal microbes formed the basis for your own distinct pattern of gut microbes, and will for the rest of your life. The mother's microbes also supply our newborns with a key piece of its metabolic machinery, giving the baby the ability to digest the milk sugars and special carbohydrates in breast milk.

Since vaginal microbes can get your newborn's intestinal tract off to a healthy start, scientists are now studying whether cesarean delivery jeopardizes a newborn's future brain health. It is amazing that in such countries as Brazil and Italy the rates of C-section delivered babies surpass those who come into this world in the natural way, even though we have no clue about the long-term consequences of "bypassing" the normal vaginally mediated gut microbiome programming on brain development. So far we know that the intestines of cesarean-born infants are colonized not by the mother's vaginal microbes, but by microbes from the mother's skin, from midwives, physicians, and nurses, and from other newborns in the maternity ward, and that important beneficial bacteria such as bifidobacteria take longer to colonize their guts than they do the guts of babies born vaginally. We know the dangerous gut microbe *Clostridium difficile* is more likely to overgrow in the gut and harm C-section babies, and that C-section babies are more likely to become obese as they get older. Scientists suspect that C-section birth may also make a child more vulnerable to brain-gut changes and serious brain disorders, including autism, and several studies are under way to find out for sure. And finally, we know from a landmark study by M. Blazer's group in mice that the transient disturbances of the gut microbiota in early life by low doses of antibiotics can have long-lasting effects on the vulnerability of adults to the detrimental results of a high-fat diet on obesity.

Adapted for Survival

Survival of the species is one of the dogmas of evolution, and nature has programmed every species to deliver it. That's how we and our animal forebears have survived for millions of years. In this chapter, I've described several mechanisms by which early life stress can influence brain and behavior of animals and humans, and have focused on our growing understanding of how stressful environments and stressed mothers imbue long-lasting changes in their baby's brain. Using different biological pathways and mechanisms, these changes program his or her stress-response system for a dangerous world. By interacting with her child, a mother modifies the salience system in her infant's brain so that the baby's gut feelings are biased in a way to be prepared for a potentially dangerous world when he or she has grown up. She alters the microbes in her vagina, changing her infant's gut microbiome. She tags key stress-response genes with chemicals called methyl groups, providing epigenetic changes that can last for several generations.

Why would evolution have developed a system that makes us unhealthy and unhappy? If nature, in its wisdom, devised several strategies toward a single end, and if those strategies can be seen in many species, including us humans, they must be there for a good reason.

The science all points in one direction. When the mother perceives danger, these strategies inculcate into her baby a heightened fight-or-flight response, plus more careful, less aggressive, and less outgoing behaviors. Even without her knowledge, she's preparing her baby for a world she perceives as dangerous.

This system may have helped us when we had to flee attacking lions or vanquish a competitor in a fistfight, as our ancient ancestors did. Even though no scientific data is available to prove this hypothesis, it may even make millions of people today who are unfortunate enough to have to face battles, famines, and natural disasters, or who grow up in rough neighborhoods, more resilient and better adapted to deal with their hostile living conditions.

But those of us in relatively safe, industrialized societies pay a high price for these ancient and inborn biological programs. As we've seen, an overactive fight-or-flight system with constantly elevated stress hormones circulating through our bodies can lead to serious mental illness, including anxiety disorders, panic disorders, and depression. It can also cause a nasty assortment of stress-sensitive physical disorders, including obesity, metabolic syndrome, heart attacks, and strokes. And finally, the hyperresponsiveness of the brain-gut axis associated with this programming can cause chronic gut disorders like irritable bowel syndrome and chronic abdominal pain.

We don't yet know whether a pregnant woman should worry if she deals with commuter traffic, project deadlines, and financial worries, and works until a few days before she's due. And we don't yet know the degree to which practices that alter the vaginal microbiome, such as antimicrobials before and during delivery, birth by cesarean section, or a young mother's diet and stress, jeopardize a child's health. We also don't know whether the huge changes we've made to our babies' early lives help explain the meteoric rise of autism, obesity, and other diseases over the last half century. However, it is clear that certain types of stress during pregnancy, and familial distress during the time when our children grow up, are harmful for their brain development and carry a high risk of permanently altering the architecture of their brain-gut-microbiome axis. I feel strongly that any interference with the normal programming of the infant's gut microbiome through avoidable stress, nonvaginal delivery, unnecessary use of antibiotics, and unhealthy dietary habits during the pre- and postnatal periods can lay the groundwork for brain-gut disorders. And the changes to the child's brain-gut axis may not be noticeable until later in life, when it may be too late to reverse them. Becoming aware of these connections and understanding the basic biological mechanisms is the first step. Implementing strategies to minimize these unhealthy influences is often more difficult. However, adhering to a healthy diet, practicing simple stress-reduction techniques during pregnancy, and being vigilant to avoid unnecessary antibiotic exposure are all options most mothers are able to consider.

New Therapies for Brain-Gut Disorders

We now know that from the time a fetus is in the womb, the stress level experienced by her mom can alter her susceptibility to stress, gut diseases, anxiety disorders, and depression. And this early life programming is not limited to maternal behaviors. We also know that any event that's a major threat to a child's well-being can alter susceptibility to the same conditions.

All of these findings can help us to understand the roots of Jennifer's health problems. Recall that when she was still in her mother's womb, her maternal grandmother was diagnosed with breast cancer, precipitating great grief and anxiety in her pregnant mother. When Jennifer was a young child and needed a nurturing family environment, her parents fought bitterly. When Jennifer was eight, her parents divorced. A large number of patients with IBS report early life stress, and Jennifer had it in spades. Such stress most likely upped her odds of developing anxiety, depression, and GI symptoms as an adult. The fact that both her mother and grandmother suffered stress-sensitive syndromes similar to hers further increased her vulnerability to develop those symptoms as well, presumably through genetic or epigenetic mechanisms or both.

These days, when I meet a patient like Jennifer who has chronic stress-related symptoms, including anxiety or IBS, I base my advice on the evolving science of brain-gut interactions as discussed in this chapter. "Your early experiences almost certainly played a role in the development of your symptoms," I say, "both in terms of your gut symptoms, as well as your anxiety and depression." I want to make sure that the patient understands the biological nature of her symptoms—that it's not just "in their head," as other doctors might have said. "But if it has all been hardwired during my first years of life, and if my family history further increases the odds that I will suffer from these symptoms, does that mean I have to live with this pain for the rest of my life?" Jennifer asked me, somewhat distressed. I told her that the bad news is that her brain-gut axis had been programmed for life, but the good news is that humans have a very unique part of the brain, the prefrontal cortex, which gives us the ability to override the function of altered brain circuits and learn new behaviors.

There are several therapies that help us to learn these new

behaviors, much as adding some new code—a patch—to an existing computer program can override the flaws in the program. Such therapies include a short course of cognitive behavioral therapy, hypnosis, or another mind-body intervention such as mindfulness-based stress reduction. Not only do these strategies ease brain-gut symptoms, such as those of irritable bowel syndrome, but they also often help treat associated symptoms of depression and anxiety. And there's more good news from recent research. These approaches can actually change the wiring of our brains, thereby helping the prefrontal cortex exert some control on an overactive emotional brain network. They can also help to reset the brain salience system, improving the way we appraise potentially threatening situations. Sometimes these mind-based approaches require a little help from the often-maligned psychotropic medications, in particular different types of antidepressants that have shown beneficial effects in mouse models of early life stress. My initial treatment plan almost always includes very low doses of tricyclic antidepressants like Elavil or similar drugs that help calm the firestorm in their limbic system in early stages of therapy. The same drugs can reduce abdominal pain with minimal side effects, and without any effects on mood or mental state. And, if appropriate for the patient, full doses of modern antidepressants, including SSRIs, can ease anxiety and depression and stabilize mood. These drugs by themselves provide significant benefit in about 30 percent of patients, but the success rate is much higher when combined with other, nonpharmacological treatments.

Based on our new scientific insights into the role of gut microbiota in the altered brain-gut interactions, I also told Jennifer to increase her intake of probiotics. Beneficial microbes such as lactobacilli and bifidobacteria delivered via fermented foods, yogurts, or in probiotic capsules may improve the diversity of the gut microbial ecosystem. In addition to naturally occurring probiotics in fermented foods, I recommend a trial of a small number of probiotics that have proven beneficial in clinical trials.

In the end, Jennifer agreed to the integrative therapy approach I recommended to her, which included a short course of cognitive behavioral therapy, including instructions in self-relaxation and self-hypnosis. She switched to a diet high in fermented foods and supplementary probiotics, and added the low dose of the antidepressant Elavil to her long-term Celexa intake. I emphasized to her that she'd probably need both the medications and nonpharmacological therapies to get better, but if she followed the treatment plan there was a good chance that she could ease off the drugs within a year.

Jennifer's symptoms didn't disappear completely. But several months later, when she returned to my clinic for a follow-up visit, she reported a 50 percent improvement of her quality of life and overall well-being, and much less frequent abdominal pain, long periods of nearly normal bowel movements, and far less anxiety. Before leaving my office, she shook my hand and with tears in her eyes said, "I wish someone had explained to me all of these connections much earlier, in particular the fact that my rough early life set me up for anxiety, depression, and IBS." Jennifer is not the only patient who has left my office telling me that.

In a sense, people like Jennifer have adapted perfectly to the stressful world of their youth, with their brains, guts, and even their gut microbes programmed in multiple ways for danger. If more doctors knew this, they'd help, rather than frustrate, patients with IBS and many other stress-related disorders. And if more patients knew this, they would find help faster and have more peace of mind.

But early life programming affects us all. Our mothers instinctively and biologically programmed us for survival, beginning when we were still in the womb. Later, our families did the best they could to steer us through a complex world. All this leaves us with a lasting trace on our basic emotional makeup, and influences how we cope, how we make decisions, and possibly our personality. By understanding how this natural programming operates, and by learning how to patch any maladapted software, we can avoid overreactions that no longer serve us, if they ever did.

A NEW UNDERSTANDING
OF EMOTIONS

From our earliest days, emotions have colored our thoughts and influenced our decisions. When danger looms, emotions help you fight or flee; they fuel the drives that help you find a partner, and they help you bond with your children. Emotions create your tastes, influence your health, foster pet peeves, and inflame your passions. Emotional feelings are quintessential to what makes us human.

As philosophers, psychologists, and, later, neuroscientists investigated emotion over the centuries, they devised increasingly sophisticated theories to explain how emotions arise, pinning their origin to the mind, the brain, or the body. But over the last few years, scientific data has emerged suggesting that they may be influenced by a source almost nobody had expected. These revolutionary findings suggest that the microbiota in our gut play a critical role in the complex interactions between mind, brain, and gut. This exciting line of research has inspired paradigm-breaking ideas regarding the role of these invisible creatures in our gut reactions and gut feelings, and how they may affect our mood, minds, and thoughts.

Can Your Gut Microbes Change Your Brain?

When I first examined Lucy, a sixty-six-year-old woman, several years ago, her medical problems didn't seem particularly unusual. For many years she had been suffering from mild constipation and discomfort in her belly, and she had been given a diagnosis of irritable bowel syndrome. What made Lucy's story so curious was her anxiety symptoms. By the time she came under my care, she'd been suffering from severe panic attacks every few weeks for two years. The symptoms included intense fear, heart palpitations, shortness of breath, and a sense of doom. These symptoms came on suddenly and usually subsided within twenty minutes. In the periods between these dramatic attacks, she had noticed, her general anxiety level had also increased. While many of the patients who see me for their gastrointestinal symptoms report a history of panic attacks, the circumstances surrounding the onset of Lucy's symptoms were highly unusual.

About two years ago she developed chronically recurring sinus congestion and headaches, and she was diagnosed with a sinus infection. While taking a two-week course of ciprofloxacin, a commonly used broad-spectrum antibiotic that kills a wide variety of pathogens (as well as our own gut microbes), she noticed that her bowel movements had become more frequent and looser, though she was fine otherwise. To counter these effects, she took probiotics for a couple of weeks and once again felt like her usual self.

About six months later, the same symptoms of congestion and headaches recurred. Her physician prescribed an alternate broad-spectrum antibiotic, which she took for three weeks. Again she experienced similar chronic discomfort in her belly. So far, none of this was out of the ordinary: many patients develop a transient change in their bowel habits when taking antibiotics because the medications temporarily suppress the diversity of gut microbes that are essential for optimal gut function. We know from patient reports and clinical studies that these side effects can include prolonged gastrointestinal discomfort and sometimes even IBS-like symptoms. In the great majority of patients, however, these GI problems are temporary. It appears that patients who start out with less diverse microbiota are more susceptible to these side effects.

Since Lucy was no longer taking antibiotics, I encouraged her to eat and drink a wide variety of fermented foods of all types, including yogurt, sauerkraut, and kimchi, and to take additional probiotic supplements as well. The goal was to increase the diversity of her gut microbiota in the hope to reestablish her original microbial architecture. At the same time, I strongly encouraged her to use approaches aimed at relieving her anxiety symptoms, including self-relaxation techniques, deep abdominal breathing, and mindfulness classes. I also prescribed Klonopin, a Valium-like medication that dissolves under the tongue, to be taken if and when Lucy began to experience a full-blown panic attack. This combined treatment regimen gradually normalized her bowel movements, and over a six-month period, her panic attacks became less frequent. When I last saw her, she had experienced only a single, mild attack, and she no longer needed to take the Klonopin.

Lucy's panic attacks and her increased anxiety had developed several weeks after her GI symptoms, and they became less frequent when her digestive symptoms improved. I suspected that the two consecutive courses of broad-spectrum antibiotics she took may have temporarily altered the population and function of her gut microbiota. This would have led to her IBS-like GI symptoms, which disappeared shortly after stopping the medication. Could the antibiotic have induced gut microbial changes that contributed to her anxiety symptoms as well?

Are Gut Microbiota Our Own Xanax Factory?

With the exception of a few clinical case reports, there was little science to support a connection between our gut microbiota and emotional states when I saw Lucy in my clinic in 2011. But later that year a group of pioneering investigators in Canada reported some intriguing findings from animal experiments that suggested that gut microbes themselves produce neurotransmitters that could change emotional behavior.

Premysl Bercik and his group at McMaster University had treated a group of normal mice for a week with a cocktail consisting of three broad-spectrum antibiotics. They monitored the mice's gut microbiota composition and their behavior before, during, and after the antibiotic treatment. As they expected, the treatment profoundly altered the makeup of the animals' gut microbial populations, increasing populations of some groups of microbes (in particular several species of lactobacilli) and decreasing populations of others. However, Bercik was surprised to see that the antibiotic-treated mice engaged in more exploratory behavior, such as spending more time in the well-lit, open areas of their cages or experimental setups rather than the dark and protected locations they usually prefer. Since mice can't tell us about their anxiety symptoms, this behavior is used as a proxy that indicates that the animals are less anxious, or as scientists say, that they showed less "anxiety-like behaviors."

Two weeks after the mice had completed the antibiotic course, both their behavior and their gut microbiota returned to their normal state, suggesting that the observed changes in the animals' emotional behavior and the antibiotic-induced changes in their gut microbiota were related. But how was the brain informed about the antibiotic-induced changes in the gut? An obvious candidate for such gut microbe-to-brain signaling was the vagus nerve, the main communication highway between the gut and the brain. And indeed, mice in which the vagus nerve was cut no longer showed the reduction in anxiety when their microbes were suppressed by the antibiotic. These findings suggested that in normal mice, gut microbes produced a steady supply of substances that were able to suppress anxiety, and their effect was transmitted to the brain through the vagus nerve.

What substances might the gut microbes produce that have such an anxiolytic effect? Previous studies had shown that certain microorganisms are able to produce the neurotransmitter gamma-aminobutyric acid. This substance, also referred to as GABA, is one of the most abundant signaling molecules in the nervous system, where it keeps the emotional part of our brain, the limbic system, in check. Many of our antianxiety medications, such as Valium, Xanax, and Klonopin, target the same signaling system, mimicking the effects of GABA.

Earlier clues about the connection between gut microbes, GABA, and brain function had been observed some thirty years ago in patients with advanced liver cirrhosis; such patients' mental status and alertness are commonly impaired. When they are given a drug that blocks the GABA signaling system, cognitive function and energy level improve rapidly. Surprisingly, brain function also improved when they received broad-spectrum antibiotics. At the time, investigators had not been able to explain well how cirrhosis of the liver could increase GABA activity in the brain. But today we know that the increased GABA produced in the gut by altered microbes finds its way to the specific GABA receptors in the brain, where it dampens cognitive processes as well as emotional brain systems. Just like in Bercik's mouse experiments, broad-spectrum antibiotics reduce the populations of these GABA-producing bacteria, leading to lower GABA levels in the brain and improved brain function.

While these experiments have clearly established the fact that microbes living in our gut can produce antianxiety molecules, and that these substances can affect the brain under certain circumstances, the great majority of patients who receive antibiotics show no evidence of emotional side effects. But could we use this knowledge to treat anxiety disorders with GABA-producing microbes, in the form of probiotics? We know that certain strains of two of the best-studied families of beneficial gut bacteria, the lactobacilli and the bifidobacteria, have the synthetic machinery to produce GABA. Since different strains of bacteria from these two families are active ingredients in most commercially available probiotics, and both groups also tend to be abundant in fermented food products, is it possible that adding an extra supply of these microbes to our diet makes us more relaxed? Could a regimen as simple as eating fermented foods and taking probiotics help anxiety-prone individuals reduce their anxiety levels? A small number of studies performed in mice suggest that this may indeed be the case. In one study, investigators observed a decrease in anxiety-like behavior when they fed the probiotic *Lactobacillus rhamnosus* to healthy adult mice. In another study, a different probiotic species, *Lactobacillus longum*, was found to decrease anxiety-like behaviors markedly in mice with colitis, a chronic inflammation of the large intestine. And there is some clinical evidence suggesting that such "psychobiotic" effects can be achieved in patients.

The only reliable way to evaluate the possible effect of probiotics on the human brain is to perform a controlled clinical trial on human subjects. In such a trial, volunteers are randomly assigned to either a group that ingests the active treatment—a probiotic, for example—or to a control group. Those in the control group ingest a placebo—a food that is indistinguishable from the treatment in appearance, taste, or flavor, but that has no known intrinsic action. To increase the reliability of such a study, neither the study participants nor the investigators are allowed to know until after the study is completed which treatment group a subject was assigned to. Such blinded, randomized, controlled study designs are the gold standard in assessing the effectiveness of all treatments in medicine.

In 2013, Kirsten Tillisch used such a study design at our research center and randomly assigned thirty-six women to one of three experimental groups. Twice a day for four weeks, the active-treatment group ate yogurt enriched with a particular strain of the probiotic *Bifidobacterium lactis*, along with three other types of bacteria (*Streptococcus thermophiles, Lactobacillus bulgaricus,* and *Lactococcus lactis*) that are typically used to turn milk into yogurt. A second group ate a nonfermented milk product that had no probiotics but was indistinguishable in taste, texture, or appearance from the probiotic-enriched yogurt. A third group ate no yogurt or milk product at all.

At the beginning and end of the four-week study, we asked each woman about her overall well-being, mood, level of anxiety, and bowel habits. Then Tillisch scanned each woman's brain as she lay in an MRI scanner and performed a task designed to test her ability to assess other people's emotions from their facial expressions.

The task consisted of watching the faces of three different people who looked angry, scared, or sad, and quickly identifying which two of the three faces displayed the same emotion, by simply pushing a button. People around the world, regardless of race, country, or language, are extremely good at making such assessments in a fraction of a second, suggesting that this is a very basic, inborn emotional reflex response that is likely related to the emotional reflex behavior of animals. The task does not involve the complex brain networks needed to generate emotional feelings, so subjects don't feel sad or angry doing the task.

Compared with women who ate the milk product with no probiotics, women who received the probiotic mix for four weeks showed less connectivity between a number of brain regions during the emotion recognition task. These results showed for the first time that some of the astonishing results from mouse studies apply to humans as well—specifically, that manipulating gut microbiota could measurably change human brain function during a task related to emotions, at least at a very basic emotional reflex level.

But how did the probiotic bacteria from the yogurt communicate with our subjects' brains? We initially thought that the regular intake of the probiotics may alter the gut microbial composition, which in turn may have an influence on the brain. However, when we analyzed the microbial composition in the stool of study participants, there were no detectable effects of the probiotic ingestion on the types and numbers of the gut microbiota, other than the presence of the ingested probiotic organism itself. Thus the yogurt consumption didn't change the players among the gut microbiota. However, based on an earlier study, we knew that the identical probiotic treatment can change the metabolites that the gut microbes produce. It is therefore reasonable to speculate that some of these probiotic-stimulated metabolites reached the brain—either via the bloodstream or in the form of a vagal nerve signal—to change the emotional reactivity of the brain. There may even be an involvement of the gut's serotonin-containing cells in this microbe-brain communication. It has recently been shown that certain gut microbes can stimulate the production of serotonin in these cells, altering serotonin levels in the gut and profoundly influencing the availability of this gut-brain signal to modulate our emotions, pain sensitivity, and well-being. If confirmed, the implications of these findings for the future treatment of brain-gut disorders are truly amazing. By consuming certain types of probiotics—either contained in naturally fermented foods or enriched in dairy products or fruit juices—that can regulate levels of the vital neurotransmitter serotonin, we may be able to fine-tune a control system in our body that plays such a crucial role in many of our vital functions, ranging from mood to pain sensitivity and sleep.

As our study subjects were carefully selected to be healthy, without any evidence of physical or psychological symptoms, we can only speculate if the changes we observed with the particular probiotic we evaluated might have affected their anxiety levels. However, as subjects showed a reduced responsiveness of emotional brain networks when paying attention to angry, sad, and fearful faces, we know that certain probiotics are able to dampen emotional reactions to negative contexts.

I was amazed at these findings. Just a few years ago, few would have thought that regular consumption of a yogurt that you can buy in the supermarket could influence your brain. For our research team, the results opened up a completely new way of looking at how our brains function in health and disease—and how to keep our minds healthy.

It is only in the last few years that scientists have begun to investigate the role of nutrition in brain health, and to identify a possible role of the gut microbiota in this relationship. Based on the rapidly advancing science of this field, I am convinced that this new perspective will profoundly change our concepts of which foods are beneficial to our emotional and mental well-being. And it may influence the way we treat anxiety disorders and depression in the future.

The Role of the Microbiota in Depression

If you've ever been depressed, you probably recall how sad, discouraged, and hopeless you felt. Those are the symptoms we usually talk about when describing depression to friends and family, and it's a painful state of affairs. But perhaps you can also recall some other symptoms. Were you nervous or irritable? Did you have a hard time sleeping or concentrating? These are the same symptoms a person with an anxiety disorder develops. Nearly half of the people diagnosed as depressed have symptoms of anxiety, and many chronically anxious people have symptoms of depression. And therapies for depression—particularly the medications known as selective serotonin reuptake inhibitors, or SSRIs—often ease the anxiety symptoms as well. The two disorders are close cousins.

Since various manipulations of the gut microbiota in mice, including the ingestion of probiotics, can ease anxiety-like behavior of these animals, might they ease the mouse equivalent of depression as well? John F. Cryan, a psychiatrist from University College, in Cork, Ireland, has published several papers supporting this hypothesis, coining the catchy term *melancholic microbes* to refer to these mood-altering properties of gut microorganisms.

However, until recently, this hypothesis derived from studies in laboratory mice was not supported by much data from human patients. There are now three well-controlled studies performed in patients with a psychiatric diagnosis of major depressive disorder that clearly implicate a role of altered gut microbes in the symptoms of depression. Patients could be classified as suffering from depression simply by looking at the composition of their gut microbiota. Even more surprising, when fecal samples containing the altered gut microbiome were transferred into either germ-free laboratory mice or rats in which the normal microbiota had been wiped out by broad spectrum antibiotic treatment, the recipient animals developed behaviors that indicated to the investigators a change in their mood, so-called "depression-like" behaviors. So clearly, the microbes living in the gut of depressed patients were able to send signals to the brain of these laboratory rodents, which changed their emotion generating brain networks resulting in a distinct emotional behavior. Even though these remarkable results have gotten us much closer to corroborate the concept of "melancholic microbes," there is still the big question: Does the brain of a depressed patient send signals to the gut that changes the composition and function of the gut microbes, or do the microbes of depressed patients play a causative role in the patients' symptoms. If the second hypothesis is correct, changing the signals the gut microbes send to the brain by the consumption of a probiotic or a particular diet could alleviate depression symptoms.

Cryan's team tested this hypothesis in the laboratory by giving laboratory rats the probiotic bacteria *Bifidobacterium infantis*, so named because it's one of the first bacterial strains a new mother transmits to her infant. They then made the rats swim, which these animals dislike and which activates their stress system. When this happens, blood levels of cytokines, a type of inflammatory molecule, climb (the same response happens in humans). When the rats were given a probiotic, it seemed to moderate the changes in both their blood and their brain, although it did not alter the animals' "depressed" behavior. In another study, the researchers were able to show that a particular strain of *Bifidobacterium* reduced experimentally induced depression and anxiety-like behavior in mice as much as the commonly used antidepressant medication Lexapro.

Do these result suggest that probiotics be helpful in human depression as well? Preliminary results suggest that this may be the case in some depressed individuals. In a randomized, blinded study, French investigators gave fifty-five healthy men and women a monthlong regimen of a daily probiotic containing species of lactobacillus and bifidobacteria. Those in the probiotic group showed a small improvement in psychological distress and anxiety compared to those taking the control product. In another study, British researchers gave a different lactobacillus species to 124 healthy people. In people who were more depressed when the study began, the treatment significantly improved their mood. There is now also new evidence that a dietary intervention known to positively affect the gut microbiome may have a beneficial effect in the treatment of depression. A recent randomized controlled study performed by Felice Jacka in Australia in patients with moderate to severe depression evaluated the possible benefit of nutritional counseling compared to social support. Nutritional counseling about the benefits of a Mediterranean diet in addition to traditional psychological or pharmacological treatment showed a statistically significant benefit to the group that received social support.

While these studies are a good start, we need bigger and better-designed clinical trials to firmly establish whether probiotic microorganisms can cheer you up if you're depressed, calm you down when you're anxious, or affect your mental well-being. In the meantime, you can positively influence your brain-gut-microbiota dialogue by paying more attention to what you feed your gut microbes. As we will learn in greater detail in subsequent chapters, what we eat has a major impact on gut health, giving us an easy, enjoyable, and inexpensive way to modify and improve our gut-brain interactions.

The Role of Stress

Most patients with anxiety disorders, depression, IBS, or other brain and brain-gut disorders are particularly sensitive to stressful events, often experiencing a flare-up of GI symptoms when they're under stress. Today we know that gut microbes play a major role in determining the responsiveness of the brain's stress circuits. We also know that the mediators of our stress system, such as the stress hormone norepinephrine, can profoundly alter gut microbial behavior, making them more aggressive and dangerous.

One of the first clues as to the possible influence of gut microbes on our emotions arose from experiments on so-called germ-free mice, and the majority of published studies about gut microbes and the brain have relied on this approach. Unlike animals raised under normal conditions, who are exposed to microbes from food, air, the people that look after them, and their own feces, germ-free animals are born and bred in completely aseptic conditions—environments with no microbes at all. Scientists breed germ-free mice by delivering baby mice by cesarean section, then immediately transferring them to isolated spaces where all incoming air, food, and water are sterilized. After these animals grow up in this sterile world, scientists study their behavior and biology and compare them to genetically identical animals raised under normal conditions. Behaviors or brain biochemistry that differ between the two groups of animals can then be considered to be dependent on normal gut microbiota.

Not long after these animals were first bred, investigators observed that as adults they overrespond to stressful stimuli by producing more of the stress hormone corticosterone (as mentioned earlier, it's the rat equivalent of cortisol, the human stress hormone). When the researchers transplanted beneficial microbiota into these animals' guts at an early age, they could reverse the exaggerated response to stress. However, such a beneficial effect of gut microbial treatment was no longer observed when given to the adult animals. These experiments revealed that gut microbes can influence the development of the brain's stress response at an early age.

If you take a litter of mice, separated them at birth into two groups, and raise one of the groups germ-free, the two groups of siblings differ in a surprisingly wide range of measures. The germ-free mice are less sensitive to pain and less social when interacting with their peers. In addition, biochemical and molecular mechanisms in the brain and in the gut are altered compared with normal mice. For example, Sven Pettersson's research group at the Karolinska Institute, in Sweden, showed that germ-free mice showed less anxiety-like behavior than normally raised animals, as well as altered expression of genes involved in nerve-cell-signaling brain regions implicated in motor control and anxiety-like behavior. But when the germ-free mice were exposed to gut microbiota early in life, they displayed none of these abnormal biochemical abnormalities. Pettersson and his colleagues concluded that when gut microbiota colonize the gut, it somehow initiates the biochemical signaling mechanisms in the brain that affect emotional behavior.

We have known for some time that different types of stress can temporarily alter gut microbial composition, specifically decreasing the number of lactobacilli in the stool of stressed animals. This was confirmed in a recent study in which laboratory mice undergoing different types of stresses over a period of several weeks not only showed a decrease in the lactobacilli population in their gut but also developed depression-like behavior. The degree of depression like behavior was closely correlated with the amount of lactobacilli lost. This change in microbial abundance was associated with a change in the molecules these lactobacilli produced, in particular a chemical that the microbes derive from tryptophan in our diet called kynurenin. This chemical is able to induce depression-like behavior in non-stressed animals, and the investigators were able to reduce its production by feeding the animals the probiotic *Lactobacillus reuteri*. Even though awaiting confirmation of this stress-microbiome-depression connection in humans, the findings suggest that the well-known association of chronic stress with the development of depression in vulnerable individuals may involve changes in the gut microbiota.

Data coming from a different area of research suggests that the effect of stress goes beyond these temporary changes in the abundance in microbial populations. It has been known for a long time that norepinephrine, a chemical that is released during times of stress, makes your heart beat faster and your blood pressure rise. But we have learned only recently that this stress mediator can also be released into the inside of your gut, where it can directly communicate with your gut microbes. Several laboratories have shown that norepinephrine can stimulate the growth of bacterial pathogens that can cause serious gut infections, stomach ulcers, and even sepsis. In addition to the growth-promoting ability of this stress molecule, it is also able to activate genes in pathogens, making them more aggressive and increasing their odds of survival in the intestine. Certain gut microbes can even modify norepinephrine that's floating around in the gut during stress into a more powerful form, intensifying the effect of the hormone on other microbes. All of this means that catching a gut infection when you are under severe stress can land you in serious trouble.

One patient who demonstrates the clinical consequences of this relationship between stress and gut infections is Mrs. Stone, a fifty-year-old woman I saw in my clinic. Mrs. Stone had just gone through lengthy, contentious, and stressful divorce proceedings to end her twenty-five-year marriage. Her job as a business executive was highly demanding, requiring eighty-hour workweeks and lots of travel. She'd never had GI symptoms that she could recall, but she had recurrent bouts of anxiety and suffered from chronic low back pain and headaches for most of her life. Mrs. Stone was seriously stressed, and she knew it.

To give herself a break, she flew from Los Angeles to Cabo San Lucas, Mexico, for a vacation. The first two days were everything she had hoped for, and she enjoyed the peace relaxing by the hotel pool. On her third day in the scenic Baja beach town, Mrs. Smith went out to eat at a local seafood place. For the rest of the week she felt miserable, barely leaving her hotel room and battling her unrelenting symptoms of belly cramps, bloating, nausea, and diarrhea.

Mrs. Stone felt better by the time she returned to Los Angeles, but she talked with her primary care doctor anyway. He diagnosed traveler's diarrhea, a common form of gastroenteritis that's typically caused by bacteria in the local water. Mrs. Stone's symptoms had already improved by the time she saw him, and there were no infectious bacteria detectable in her stool sample, so her doctor recommended against taking an antibiotic and assured her that the symptoms would disappear completely in a few days.

Unfortunately, they didn't, and after several weeks of residual symptoms, including constant bloating, irregular bowel movements, and occasional cramps, Mrs. Stone made an appointment to see me. Since Mrs. Stone's stool tests for infectious organisms again turned out negative and she had never experienced any gastrointestinal symptoms before, I recommended a colonoscopy. When this endoscopic test turned up nothing abnormal, I diagnosed postinfectious irritable bowel syndrome.

This syndrome affects approximately 10 percent of patients with proven bacterial or viral gastroenteritis, and it occurs most often in people with previous symptoms of pain and discomfort anywhere in the body, whose initial bout of infectious gastroenteritis lasts longer than usual, and who contract their GI infection when they're experiencing chronic severe stress. (If you do contract this disease, know that symptoms typically disappear over several months, and that the syndrome is treatable with standard IBS therapies.)

Individuals with these risk factors are more likely than most to develop postinfectious IBS-like symptoms when a pathogen like enterotoxigenic *E. coli*, the most common cause of traveler's diarrhea, infects them. This makes great sense because chronic stress stimulates the growth of many pathogens, including *E. coli*, in our gut, and makes them more aggressive. It also causes the autonomic nervous system in our gut to release stress signals that can reduce the thickness of the mucus layer lining the colon wall and make your gut leakier, allowing microbes greater access to the gut's immune system by circumventing many of our gut's defensive strategies. This chain of events results in a longer-lasting intestinal immune activation and prolonged symptoms.

As we all know, not all stress is bad for us. In contrast to chronic, or recurrent stress, acute stress and its associated emotional arousal improve our performance on difficult tasks, such as taking a test or giving a talk. It also benefits gut health by strengthening our defenses to gut infections. This works in multiple ways. Acute stress increases acid production by the stomach in response to stress-related brain signals, which makes it more likely that invading microbes from our food will be killed before they reach our intestine. It also signals the intestine to increase fluid secretion and expel its contents, including the pathogen. Finally, it increases the secretion of antimicrobial peptides called defensins. All these responses are aimed at defending the integrity of the gastrointestinal tract against potentially dangerous invaders and shortening the duration of an infection.

But despite these protective effects of acute stress on our gut and its microbes, too much of it turns the benefits into a liability. Chronic stress increases your risk of developing gastrointestinal infections, and is likely to prolong your suffering of symptoms after the infection has cleared. And if you are suffering from stress-sensitive conditions like IBS or cyclical vomiting syndrome, chronic stress is one of the main drivers of symptom severity.

Positive Emotions

We know a lot about the detrimental effects of chronic stress on brain-gut-microbiome interactions. But do other emotions besides stress, in particular positive emotions, also affect the microbes in your gut? That is, does happiness or a sense of well-being elicit different, beneficial gut reactions?

We've seen how each of these emotions and their underlying operating systems in the brain can be triggered by a distinct chemical signal—endorphins when we're happy, oxytocin when we feel close to our spouse or children, and dopamine when we're longing for something. When these chemical switches trigger the respective operating systems in the brain, it leads to a distinct gut reaction with characteristic patterns of contractions, secretions, and intestinal blood flow.

I suspect that some of these gut reactions associated with positive emotions are also associated with the release of distinct chemical messages to our gut microbes. We already know that serotonin, dopamine, and endorphins are released into the gut interior, and they would be good candidates for such positive gut-to-microbe signals. This emotion-related signaling from brain to gut microbes may alter the behavior of the microbes in a way that benefits our health and protects us from gut infections. Signals associated with happiness or affection may prove to increase gut microbial diversity, improve gut health, and protect us from gut infections and other diseases.

Other Consequences of Emotions on Gut Microbes

So far, we know only a small part of this fascinating story. We are beginning to understand how gut microbes can translate information contained in the food we eat into molecular signals that influence many of our body's organs and tissues, including the brain. We already know that of the thousands of different metabolites in our bloodstream, up to 40 percent come from our gut microbes. Moreover, gut reactions to specific emotions—positive and negative ones—may dramatically alter the mix of metabolites that gut microbes produce from the food—in other words, they'll heavily edit the molecular signals our gut microbes send to the rest of our body. I expect we'll learn that those trillions of bacteria in our intestines, which scientists neglected for so many years, not only are influenced by our emotions, but also exert a powerful influence not just on our gut, but on how we think and how we feel.

Can Your Gut Microbes Alter Your Social Behavior?

If our gut microbes can affect our emotions, and emotions and gut feelings drive our decisions on how to behave, it logically follows that gut microbes can alter our behavior. And if gut microbes alter our behavior, then could an abnormal mix of gut microbes lead to abnormal behaviors? And if *that's* true, could replacing abnormal gut microbes with healthy ones improve not just intestinal problems, but behavior itself?

Jonathan and his mother believed that it just might. Jonathan was twenty-five years old when the two arrived in my clinic. He had been diagnosed with autism spectrum disorder (ASD), the current term for people on the autism spectrum, as well as obsessive-compulsive disorder and chronic anxiety. Like many people with ASD, Jonathan had always suffered from a range of gastrointestinal problems, which in his case included abdominal bloating, pain, and constipation.

Jonathan's bloating symptoms got much worse after he received several courses of broad-spectrum antibiotics, suggesting that altered gut microbiota may have played a role when his gastrointestinal symptoms flared up. Like many patients with ASD, he had already tried several diets, including a gluten-free diet and a dairy-free diet, without any lasting benefit. His unusual day-to-day diet was not helping him, either, but that wasn't surprising. He ate almost no fruits or vegetables, as he disliked both their texture and smell. Instead, his diet consisted largely of refined carbohydrates, including pancakes, waffles, potatoes, noodles, pizza, snacks, and protein bars, as well as some meat and chicken.

From surfing the Internet, Jonathan was well informed about health issues in general and about the gut microbiome in particular. He had read about the effects of bad gut bacteria and parasites on the GI system, and he was convinced that his gut symptoms were related to the evildoings of a parasite in his gut. He had recently begun cognitive behavioral therapy to treat these phobias and obsessions, and the therapy involved exposure to food he disliked. This caused him a considerable amount of anxiety and stress, and I suspected that this transient stress might have been worsening his gastrointestinal symptoms.

I requested a detailed analysis of the microbiota in his stool through the American Gut Project, a crowd-funded research project that's obtaining fecal samples from thousands of ordinary people to learn more about how diet and lifestyle shape our gut microbiota. A series of studies in recent years has suggested that patients on the autism spectrum may have an altered mix of gut microbes relative to individuals without ASD symptoms, including proportionally more of a bacteria group known as Firmicutes and less of a group called Bacteroidetes. Patients with irritable bowel syndrome exhibit a similar pattern. Jonathan's analysis revealed that he had the same pattern, and that he had fewer bacteria known as Proteobacteria and Actinobacteria than the average American. However, since he had an unusual diet, suffered from anxiety and stress, and also had IBS-like symptoms, we had no way of knowing if it was his ASD, his IBS, or his unique eating habits that were responsible for his altered mix of gut microbes.

Among other questions, Jonathan and his mother wanted to know whether Jonathan should consider undergoing a fecal microbial transplantation or take probiotics to change his microbiome to help with his psychological and gastrointestinal symptoms. They asked because news of a recent animal study had spread like wildfire through the autism community, igniting a great deal of hope in these experimental therapies.

Up to 40 percent of patients with a diagnosis of ASD suffer from gastrointestinal symptoms, mostly altered bowel habits and abdominal pain and discomfort, and many of these patients meet diagnostic criteria for irritable bowel syndrome. In addition, people with ASD have other abnormalities in their gut-microbiome-brain axis. They commonly have elevated blood levels of the brain-gut signaling molecule serotonin. (Remember that more than 90 percent of this molecule is stored in the gut and that serotonin-containing gut cells are in close communication with the vagus nerve and the brain.) And in patients with this disorder, their gut microbiota composition is altered, as are some metabolites in their blood.

In one of the best and most influential animal studies done yet, Sarkis Mazmanian and Elaine Hsiao of the California Institute of Technology (Caltech), in Pasadena, injected pregnant mice with a substance that mimics viral infection and activates their immune system. Young mice born of such mothers exhibit a range of altered behaviors that resemble those of people with ASD, including anxiety-like behavior, stereotypic repetitive behaviors, and compromised social interactions. For this reason, this so-called maternal immune activation model is a valid animal model for autism.

The Caltech investigators found that the young mice exhibited changes in their gut and the gut microbiota: an imbalanced mix of gut microbes, a leakier intestine, and greater engagement of the gut-based immune system. The investigators identified a particular gut microbial metabolite that was closely related to a metabolite that had previously been identified in the urine of children with ASD. When they gave this metabolite to healthy mice born to mothers whose immune system had not been activated, those mice had the same behavioral abnormalities as mice born to mothers whose immune systems had. Most intriguing, when they transplanted the stool of the abnormal mice into germ-free mice that behaved normally, the transplanted animals behaved abnormally. This strongly suggested that transplanted stool from the affected animals produced a metabolite that could reach the brain and alter the behavior of healthy mice. Most important for people with autism spectrum disorders, they could make several (though not all) of the autism-like behaviors disappear by treating the affected mice with human intestinal bacteria called *Bacteroides fragilis.*

This carefully designed study garnered a lot of attention and excitement not only in the scientific community, but also among parents of autistic children and among companies eager to develop novel therapies for this devastating disorder. Jonathan and his mother were among those who learned about the study, and they asked me whether Jonathan should consider undergoing a fecal microbial transplantation or taking probiotics to help with his psychological and gastrointestinal symptoms.

I explained to the patient that several ongoing studies in human patients with ASD will be able to answer his questions definitively within the next couple of years. It would be a tremendous scientific breakthrough if even a subset of affected ASD patients showed symptom improvement with such therapies. But even before these results are known, there are several things I was able to recommend to alleviate some of his symptoms. It is important to remember that there are several factors that contribute to Jonathan's gastrointestinal symptoms. First, he chooses food based on its texture rather than its taste, resulting in a highly restricted diet avoiding many plant-based foods. Second, he consumes a lot of processed food. Third, his high anxiety levels and stress sensitivity alter his gastrointestinal contractions and secretions and increase the leakiness of his gut.

My treatment plan targeted both his brain and his gut: Our dietitian worked with him to help him gradually change his diet from being highly restricted to a more balanced diet, including fruits, vegetables, and a range of fermented products (including fermented dairy products, probiotic-enriched soft drinks, kimchi, sauerkraut, different cheeses), all of which contain different species of lactobacilli and bifidobacteria. I suggested a trial of herbal laxatives, such as low doses of rhubarb root or aloe vera preparations to treat his constipation. And last but not least, we taught the patient self-relaxation exercises such as abdominal breathing and strongly recommended he continue his ongoing cognitive behavioral therapy for his phobias and increased anxiety level.

When Jonathan returned two months later his gastrointestinal symptoms were much improved. He had increased the variety of foods he was willing to eat, and he was able to have normal bowel movements. He was no longer obsessing about evil parasites in his gut, but was more interested in understanding how his diet can influence the behavior of his gut microbiota, and how this interaction could improve his GI symptoms.

Toward a New Theory of Emotions

Long before anybody knew about the complexity of gut microbes, gut sensations, and their effects on the brain, two prominent nineteenth-century scholars formulated the first comprehensive theory of emotions. The American philosopher, psychologist, and physician William James and the Danish physician Carl Lange proposed in the mid-1880s that emotions arise from our cognitive appraisal of bodily sensations—that is, interoceptive information from our organs as they engage in intense activity, such as a rapid heartbeat, a growling stomach, a spastically contracted colon, or rapid breathing. This theory, called the James-Lange theory of emotion, is famous among psychologists, though of course few people today believe that emotions arise *entirely* from bodily sensations.

In 1927, the renowned physiologist Walter Cannon, at Harvard University, refuted the James-Lange theory with an extensive body of empirical data, proposing a brain-based theory in which the activity in specific brain regions such as the amygdala and the hypothalamus responding to environmental stimuli generated the emotional experience. Even though we know now that these brain regions are in fact essential in generating emotions, Cannon did not have access to the powerful brain-imaging tools we have at our disposal today. Thus he could not have known about the chemical- and nerve-mediated feedback systems to the brain. Nor could he have had any idea about the prominent role of the gut and the gut microbes in this interoceptive system.

It was not until modern-day neuroscientists, including Antonio Damasio and Bud Craig, came up with anatomically based theories about brain-body loops composed of both sensory and executive components that the old theories were replaced by a unifying concept of how our emotions are generated and modulated.

Craig extensively studied the neuroanatomy of pathways that carry information from the body to the brain, or interoceptive information. Based on these studies, he proposed that every emotion has two closely connected components: a sensory component (including gut feelings) and an action component (including gut reactions). The sensory component is an

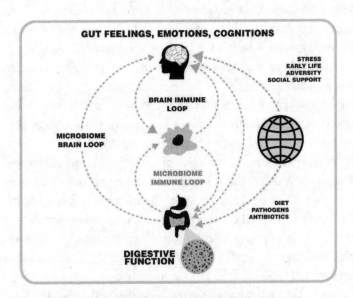

FIG. 5. THE CLOSE LINK OF THE GUT MICROBIOME-BRAIN AXIS WITH THE EXTERNAL WORLD

The gut-brain axis is not only involved in regulatory loops within the body (immune and endocrine systems) but it is also closely linked to the world around us. The brain responds to various psychosocial influences, whereas the gut and its microbiome respond to what we eat, which medications we take, and to any infectious organisms. The entire system functions like a supercomputer which integrates vast amounts of information from within our bodies and from the outside world we live in, to generate optimal digestive and brain functions.

interoceptive image of the body that forms in the insular cortex from a myriad of neuronal signals from various parts of the body, including the GI tract. This image is always linked to an action—a motor response that is sent back to the body from a different region of the brain, the cingulate cortex. This sets up a circular loop between the body and the brain. According to Craig's theory, the purpose of every emotion is to maintain balance of the entire organism.

Over the course of three books, neurologist and author Antonio Damasio elegantly formulated the somatic marker hypothesis that he introduced in *Descartes' Error: Emotion, Reason, and the Human Brain*. According to Damasio's theory, we have so-called body loops that consist of signals traveling from the brain to the body and back. This information about the body's response to an emotional state is stored as rich, unconscious memories of bodily states, such as muscle tension, rapid heartbeat, and shallow breathing. While Damasio said little in his theory about the prominent role of the GI tract in this process his pioneering work and publications fundamentally changed our biological understanding of emotions and emotional feelings.

The "hidden island" part of the brain, the insular cortex, discussed in more detail in the next chapter, can and does retrieve this somatic marker information. Our brains can retrieve the edited video clips of how we felt when we felt vivid emotions, including the motivations that drove us to respond. They can also use archived video clips from memory to create states of disgust, happiness, and craving without having to go through the lengthy brain-gut loop. Thus, when we experience an emotion as an adult, the brain does not need to feel sensations that describe what's actually happening in the body. Instead, it simply responds to a cue by accessing its library of emotional videos to generate a feeling. The videos in this library may have been recorded during infancy or adolescence as true gut reactions, for example the gut contractions associated with a feeling of anger. They're reported back to the brain as gut sensations and stored in the library as gut feelings such as nausea, well-being, satiation, hunger, and more. These gut feelings can be accessed for a lifetime, instantaneously.

It is only in the last decade that the exponential growth in our understanding of the gut microbiota and their interactions with the gut and the brain has forced us to expand these modern theories and include the gut microbiota as an essential third component in an expanded theory of emotion. This theory postulates that our basic brain-based emotional circuitry is largely genetically determined, present at birth, and epigenetically modified during early life. However, the full development of emotions and gut reactions requires an extensive lifelong learning process by which we train and fine-tune our brain-gut-microbiome system. Our unique personal development, lifestyle, and eating habits all fine-tune our emotion-generating machinery, creating a vast database in the brain that stores highly personal information.

It turns out that our gut microbiota play a critical role in this process, allowing us to generate very personalized patterns of emotions. It acts on our emotions primarily through the metabolites it produces. There are some 8 million microbial genes in the gut—400 times more than in the human genome. Even more astonishing, we humans differ very little from each other genetically, sharing more than 90 percent of our genes, but the assortment of microbial genes in our guts differs dramatically, and only 5 percent of them are shared between any two individuals. The gut microbiome adds a whole new dimension of complexity and possibilities to our brain-gut emotion-generating machinery.

As illustrated in Fig. 5, the bidirectional communication between the brain and the gut and the microorganisms living in it forces us to reevaluate the answer to the famous "chicken and egg" question: Are the microbes influencing what goes on in our brains, our feelings, and emotions, or are the signals the brain sends to the gut based on a particular emotional state influence the gut microbes? Based on what we have learned so far, both mechanisms are at play, forming a circular, reverberating communication circuit which can be triggered or modulated both from the brain or from the gut.

Because our gut microbiota appear so central to the way we sense emotion, anything that modifies the metabolic activity of the microbiota, including stress, diet, antibiotics, and probiotics, can in principle modulate the development and responsiveness of your emotion-generating circuits. For example, could the geographic differences in emotionality we see in people living in different parts of the world be related to geographic differences in diets and in gut microbial function? If the proposed new theory of emotions is correct, the answer is yes. While future studies are required to confirm such connections, we can say the following: while the basics of emotions could probably still be generated in an imaginary brain in a jar, completely isolated from the gut and the body, such a brain would have a very limited repertoire of emotional experiences. I strongly feel that it is the engagement of the gut, and its microbiome, that plays a major role in determining the intensity, duration, and uniqueness of our emotional feelings.

7

UNDERSTANDING INTUITIVE DECISION MAKING

Many of the decisions we make in life are grounded in logic, the product of thoughtful and careful consideration. On the other hand, there are those choices you make without any real analysis or considered reason. Such choices are often made without conscious awareness, as when you decide what to eat, what to wear, or what movie to watch.

In his bestselling book *Thinking, Fast and Slow*, psychologist Daniel Kahneman, co-winner of the 2002 Nobel Prize for economics, suggests that intuitive decision making is the "secret author of many of the choices and judgments [we] . . . make." The idea that you can make decisions about what is best for you based on intuition or gut feelings—as opposed to donning a rational thinking cap—is central to the human condition.

In fact, that kind of nonrational decision making has played a central role in my own life. When I was seventeen years old,

I worked after school at the family business, my parents' confectionery shop in the Bavarian Alps. It was an idyllic place to grow up, in the middle of a major skiing and hiking area, and only a few hours' drive from Italy. The shop was founded by my great-grandfather in 1887 and it had been owned and run by my family ever since. As a teenager, I made pastries and cakes for all kinds of occasions and particularly loved whipping up fancy chocolates into exotic shapes and sizes. It was there that I learned to associate certain aromas with different seasons and holidays, laying the basis (without any conscious awareness on my part) for my future career in studying the intricate dialogue between food, the gut, and the brain.

When it was time to decide about college, I agonized for months between becoming a fifth-generation confectioner or pursuing a career in science and medicine. On the one side, there were the attractions of taking over a well-established and lucrative business—staying connected to a closely knit community, living near friends and family, and being able to spend my free time in the town's beautiful landscape. There were also the expectations of my father, who had always planned that I would continue the proud family tradition. On the other hand, I felt pulled in a totally different direction: a rejection of traditions and routines, a love for reading books, in particular those dealing with psychology, philosophy, and science, and an insatiable curiosity about the scientific underpinnings of the mind. Unable to choose based on a list of pros and cons, I began for the first time in my life to listen to my gut feelings.

Ultimately, to the great disappointment of my father, I decided to leave the family business behind and begin my studies in Munich. When I finished medical school several years later, another gut-based decision pulled me even farther away from home and from the established career path of a German university professor, when I rejected a coveted residency training position at the university hospital in Munich and joined a research institute in Los Angeles, the Center for Ulcer Research and Education, known by its acronym CURE. The center had become a magnet for researchers from around the world interested in learning about the gut-brain dialogue. After the first few days in the lab, it became very clear that my new activities—purifying and testing various molecules from pig intestines we collected in the slaughterhouse—had none of the charms of the chocolate factory back home.

However, I became fascinated with my new work when I slowly realized that the implications of my research weren't limited to the gut: the identical signaling molecules we were isolating from the pig intestines were also found in the brain, and they were also used by a wide range of plants, animals, exotic frogs, and yes, even bacteria, to communicate with each other—a fact that has become known in science-speak as inter-kingdom signaling. Little did I know that this area of brain-gut communication would occupy my scientific interest for the rest of my medical career.

While my gut feelings had a profound influence on my life, the reality is that the stakes were not all that high. I was given many opportunities in those early years to explore different paths—and chances are, I could have been happy with whatever I'd chosen. But for others, gut decisions can be a matter of life and death.

On September 26, 1983, a young duty officer in the Soviet Air Defense Forces, Stanislav Petrov, was stationed in a bunker outside Moscow when Soviet satellites mistakenly detected five U.S. ballistic missiles heading toward the USSR. Even though alarm bells sounded, and a screen flashed "LAUNCH," Petrov made the monumental decision that the alarm was false and refused to confirm the incoming strike. Had he acted upon the "rational" procedures that were put in place for such a situation (like many of his military colleagues might have done), his retaliatory strike would have been followed by a U.S. retaliation, in all likelihood causing many millions of deaths.

Petrov initially gave several rational explanations for his decision, including his belief that an attack by five missiles didn't make sense. Any U.S. strike would be massive, with hundreds of missiles. Moreover, the launch detection system was new and, in his view, not yet wholly trustworthy. Finally, ground radar failed to confirm the attack.

However, in a 2013 interview, when it was safer to make such an honest statement, Petrov said he was never sure that the alarm was erroneous, but that he made his decision on "a funny feeling in my gut."

People the world over refer to gut-based decisions in a similar way. It does not seem to matter what type of decision is being made—political, personal, or professional, whom to marry, what college to attend, what house to buy. Presidents ultimately make gut-based decisions about war and peace, affecting millions of people, after they have listened to their advisors and carefully weighed the options on the table. If it's important, humans listen to their gut.

Gut feelings and intuitions can be viewed as opposite sides of the same coin. Intuition is your capacity for quick and ready insight. Often you know and understand things instantly, without rational thought or inference. You feel when something's fishy. You sense when you have an instant personal bond with a stranger. You are positive that the charismatic politician on television is lying through his teeth. Gut feelings reflect an extensive and often deeply personal body of wisdom that we have access to, and that we trust more than the advice provided by family members, highly paid advisors, and self-declared experts or social media.

So exactly what is a gut feeling? What's its biological basis?

And what role do the signals originating in the gut have in the generation of gut feelings? In other words, when does a gut sensation become an emotional feeling?

Some answers can be found in the extraordinary work of Bud Craig, a neuroanatomist who has advanced our understanding of the circuitry that allows your brain to listen to your body and vice versa. His ideas, laid out in a recent book, *How Do You Feel? An Interoceptive Moment with Your Neurobiological Self,* have played an important role in my own research, which looks at how your brain listens to your gut and the microbes that live in it (and vice versa).

The complex neurobiological process by which our brain constructs subjective gut feelings from the vast amount of information it receives in the form of gut sensations 24/7 is the foundation for the subjective experience of *how we feel* the moment we awake, after we eat a delicious meal, or endure a prolonged fast. There is growing evidence to suggest that the constant stream of interoceptive information from the gut (including the chatter of our gut microbiota) may play a crucial role in the generation of our gut feelings, thereby influencing our emotions.

Feelings (including gut feelings) are sensory signals that tap into your brain's so-called salience system. Salience is the level to which something in the environment can catch and retain one's attention, because it is important or noticeable; something that stands out. A bee buzzing around your head while you read this chapter may command more of your attention than the contents of the chapter, in particular because there is the potential threat of the bee stinging you. A thunderstorm outside may have similar salience and be equally effective to focus your attention away from the book, while background music playing at a low volume, or the sounds of a gentle breeze outside, may go unnoticed. The brain's salience system appraises the relevance of any signal regardless of whether it comes from

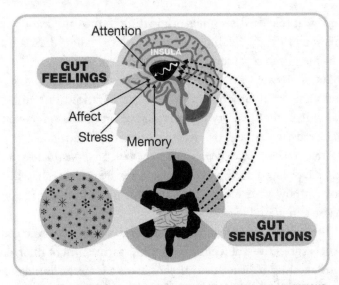

FIG. 6. HOW THE BRAIN CONSTRUCTS GUT FEELINGS FROM GUT SENSATIONS

Signals arising from the gut and its microbiome, including chemical, immune, and mechanical signals, are encoded by a vast array of receptors in the gut wall and sent to the brain via nerve pathways (in particular the vagus nerve) and via the bloodstream. This information in its raw format is received in the back portion of the insular cortex and then processed and integrated with many other brain systems. We only become aware of a small portion of this information in the form of gut feelings. Even though they originate in the gut, gut feelings are created from the integration of many other influences, including memory, attention, and affect.

your body or from the environment, to the point where the signal enters our attentional processes and our consciousness.

High-salience events related to gut sensations (including nausea, vomiting, and diarrhea) are usually accompanied by emotional feelings of discomfort and sometimes pain, alerting us that something important is going on that requires attention and a behavioral response. However, gut feelings can also be associated with positive gut sensations, such as feeling good and satiated after a nice meal, or the pleasant sensation experienced in the pit of the stomach in a fully relaxed state. The threshold for what your brain appraises as salient is influenced by many factors, including your genes, the quality and nature of your early life experiences, your current emotional state (the more anxious you are, the lower will be the salience threshold), your mindfulness of body sensations, and your vast memories of emotional moments, acquired over a lifetime. But remember, in terms of signals originating in our digestive system, most of the time your salience system operates below the level of conscious awareness. Trillions of sensory signals rise up from your gut every day and are processed in your brain's salience network, yet most don't attract your attention. They remain below the surface, content to percolate into your subconscious.

How does the salience system decide which one of these signals becomes a consciously perceived gut feeling? One brain region that plays a crucial role in this process is the insular cortex, which is the central hub of the brain's salience network. The insula, as it is also known, was given its name because of its location as "a hidden island" beneath the temporal cortex. In a theory based on neuroscientist Bud Craig's paradigm-shifting concepts and a wealth of scientific data, different regions of this hidden island in our brain are thought to play specific roles in recording, processing, evaluating, and responding to interoceptive information. According to the current understanding of how the brain handles this tremendous task, the representation of the primary image of our body is first encoded in a netork of nuclei located in the lowest part of the brain, the so-called brainstem. From there, much of this information reaches the back part of the insulaar cortex. There our perception of this image is comparable to a grainy black-and-white picture that reflects the state of every cell in our body, yet is barely visible to the naked eye.

Actually, our brains are not really interested in our comments on this information, so this raw image is not intended for our viewing pleasure. The information contained in it is relevant mainly for routine, steady-state feedback by the brain to the body region where the information originated—in our case, the gastrointestinal tract. In theory, the National Security Agency handles data the same way. In a perfect world, no one would access any of the agency's stored information unless a salience threshold were breached, alerting security agents to scrutinize telephone, Internet, and travel patterns.

The insular image is then refined, edited, and colored, similar to the process an actor's or actress's head shot undergoes after a film shoot. What Craig calls the "re-representation" of the interoceptive image of your body into ever-more-refined image versions can be compared to the process that is used in professional photography. Like a photographer using Photoshop, the brain uses affective, cognitive, and attentional tools as well as memory databases of previous experiences to refine the quality and salience of the image. As the editing progresses, the brain's attentional networks become more engaged, causing us to become more aware of the image and associate it with motivational states—that is, a drive to do something in response to the feeling being generated. It is where your visceral sensations and gustatory experiences are sent to in your brain, allowing you to feel the need to eat or eliminate, rest or run, save energy or expend energy. Once this process reaches the frontal part of the insular cortex, the image has all the features of a conscious emotional feeling that describes the state of your whole body and that we are connecting to our sense of self: feeling well, feeling nauseated, feeling thirsty, hungry, or satiated, feeling relaxed, or simply feeling unwell. From a neurobiological viewpoint, these are our true gut feelings. Despite its central role in this process, it is important to remember that the insula doesn't handle this remarkable task in isolation, but does it in close interactions with other parts of the brain's interoceptive network. This network includes several nuclei in the brainstem and different regions of the brain's cortex.

But what does our brain do with the myriad gut feelings we have accumulated over a lifetime? It would hardly make sense that evolution has come up with such an amazingly complex data-gathering and processing system, only to throw the collected information away. This library of gut feelings is composed of an enormous amount of personal and salient information about each of us that has been collected every second of the day, 365 days a year. The current scientific thinking is that this information is stored in an exponentially growing database, analogous to data collection systems created by companies and government agencies. The data collected in our brains is about highly personal experiences, our motivational drives, and our emotional reactions to these experiences, which our brains have been constructing since birth and maybe even in utero. Even though most people have paid little attention to this process or thought about its implications, we will see that it has a great deal to do with gut-feeling-based decision making.

This stored information represents countless positive and negative emotional states that we have experienced in our lifetime. For example, emotional memories may be associated with negative outcomes of decisions we have made, such as the awful abdominal pain and discomfort I experienced in Manali. This database archives the butterflies we experience in our stomachs before a job interview, or the knot that forms in the pit of our belly when we are really angry or personally disappointed. Such markers may also be associated with the pleasure of a delicious meal or the intense feelings of romantic love, or the feeling of empowerment.

Individual Differences

Pretend you are a participant in an experiment designed to look at the relationship between interoception and emotional intelligence. You lie down in a brain scanner, put on headphones, and place your left middle finger on a pad that monitors your heart rate. Your right hand rests on another pad with two buttons. As the scanner monitors your brain activity, you listen through the headphone to several series of ten beeps. After each ten-beep sequence there is a pause and you are asked to make a choice: press one button if you think the beeps were in time with your own heartbeats, or press the other button if you think the beeps were slightly out of sync with your heart. You will hear these sequences repeated, sometimes in sync, sometimes not. Can you tell the difference?

When this experiment was carried out several years ago on nine women and eight men, four subjects were supremely confident about when the pulse was synchronous or asynchronous with their hearts. They could feel the difference, accurately, every time. Two subjects were veritably heart blind. They never had a clue about whether the pulses were in or out of sync, and could only guess at random. The others fell in between.

Brain scans revealed significant activity in several brain regions of all of the participants, notably the right frontal insula. It showed the greatest activity in those who were best at following their heartbeats. Most important, these were the people who scored highest on a standardized questionnaire to probe their empathy levels. So the better you are at tracking your own heartbeats, the better you are at experiencing the full gamut of human emotions and gut feelings. The more viscerally aware, the more emotionally attuned you are. Even though this study was done with a focus on sensations from the heart, there is no reason to doubt that it would equally apply to the awareness of gut sensations.

Early Development

Gut feelings and moral intuitions have an interesting origin, related to, of all things, food. Hunger is an early emotion related to survival. And it is foundational to all the gut feelings you experience later in life, including your sense of right and wrong.

Let me explain with a story. My wife and I recently hosted some close friends for the weekend, along with their adult daughter and seven-month-old granddaughter, Lyla, who babbled most of the day. The baby was happy much of the time, but her smile and obviously good mood were interrupted whenever she got hungry, tired, or was about to fall asleep. We now know that the gut-brain axis at age seven months is a work in progress, particularly in terms of full brain development and the salience network. Moreover, gut microbes are not fully established until the end of the third year of life. Still, Lyla's primitive salience network was tuned to gut sensations related to hunger and this led to lusty crying that got her the milk she wanted. Once she was fed, Lyla's initial aversive gut feeling was quickly replaced by one of comfort and pleasure, triggered by new gut sensations related to satiation.

My main point: gut feelings related to hunger comprise your earliest signals about what is good and bad in the world, and they begin at birth. The gut feeling of an empty stomach may be a newborn child's first negative proto-emotion, triggering an uncontrollable craving for food. Similarly, the satiated feeling that follows the consumption of breast milk—which is full of prebiotics and probiotics—is likely the earliest experience of feeling good. Other positive gut feelings include gentle touch (part of interoception) with Mom, as well as warmth and comforting sound.

The signals sent from your gut to your brain, the gut sensations, play a key part in these early experiences and, by extension, your ability to differentiate good from bad. When your stomach was empty, it released a hormone, ghrelin, that led to an urgent feeling of hunger. This sensation, coupled with a strong motivational drive, would be the basis of other bad gut feelings.

Gut feelings can also be associated with positive sensations, such as the warmth of feeling full after a good meal, the pleasant sensation in the pit of your stomach while practicing abdominal breathing, or smelling chocolate aromas in a family confectionery.

The cycling experience in infancy of feeling full or hungry—good or bad—may lay the foundation for the moral judgments of good and bad that emerge into gut feelings later in life. In other words, your gut registered how well your needs were met or not met in infancy. A hungry baby left in its crib to cry for an hour perceives the world very differently from the baby who is quickly picked up, cradled, and fed. Thus your earliest gut feelings serve as a model for "what the world is like and what I must do to survive in it."

Sigmund Freud intuited as much when he developed his pragmatic understanding of primary motivational forces. The great psychiatrist linked psychological and character development to the infant's fixation on the "entry and exit" regions of the digestive tract—his famous "oral" and "anal" phases of psychic development. But Freud missed the crucial contribution of feelings, constructed by the brain based on sensory information coming from the entire digestive tract and its resident microbes—something we are only now beginning to appreciate.

How do the vast assemblies of gut microbes contribute to these early feelings of "good" and "bad"? Recall that your body is host to trillions of microbes that outnumber all of the human cells in your body. They live pretty much everywhere—on your skin, between your teeth, in saliva, in your stomach, and—most relevant to gut feelings—in your gastrointestinal tract. Your gut is home to more than a thousand microbial species that are, at multiple levels, talking to your brain.

Based on emerging evidence about the development of the gut microbial ecology during the first three years of life, we can make some intriguing speculations. It's plausible from animal studies that gut microbes influence the emotional state and development of infants the world over, from crying to cooing.

How? Some of it has to do with mother's milk, which contains something akin to Valium. The gut microbes in all infants are adapted to optimally metabolize the complex carbohydrates in breast milk. One of the microbes best suited for this is a certain strain of lactobacillus that makes a metabolite of GABA—a substance that acts on the same brain receptors as the anxiety-reducing drug Valium. By producing endogenous Valium, a microbe may help to calm down babies' emotion-generating system in the brain, and make them feel good by relieving them of hunger pangs.

Human breast milk also contains complex sugars that are not only essential for the baby's developing gut microbiome, but may also contribute to a baby's sense of well-being when it's fed. When newborn rats are fed sugar water, sweet-taste receptors in the gut and mouth generate sensations that are processed by the brain. These lead to the release of endogenous opioid molecules that reduce pain sensitivity, and presumably make rodents feel pretty good. The same may be true for human infants.

What Makes Our Brains
Uniquely Human

In all the talk about what makes humans special, you'll hear many of the same arguments. We walk upright. We have opposable thumbs. Our brains are enormous. We have language. We're top predators. But there are two features of our brains that are most relevant to our discussion about gut feelings and intuitive decision making.

The size and complexity of the frontal insula region and the closely connected prefrontal cortex—the hub of the salience network and the site where our gut feelings are created, stored, and retrieved—is what most distinguishes us from all other species. The animals closest to us in terms of relative size of their anterior insula are some of our simian cousins, in particular certain species of gorillas, followed by whales, dolphins, and elephants—all widely recognized for their emotional, social, and cognitive brain capabilities and, not coincidentally, their Animal Planet popularity.

However, there is another feature particular to the human brain that you've probably never heard about. Tucked into your right frontal insula and its associated structures lies a special class of cell found in no other species except great apes, elephants, dolphins, and whales. Called von Economo neurons (or briefly VENs), after the scientist who first observed them in 1925, they are big, fat, highly connected neurons that appear to be in the catbird seat for enabling you to make fast, intuitive judgments.

You can make snap judgments because your brain contains VENs, but to keep things simple, let's call them intuition cells. A very small number of intuition cells showed up in your brain a few weeks before you were born. Studies suggest that you probably had about 28,000 such cells at birth and 184,000 by the time you were four years old. By the time you reached adulthood, you had 193,000 intuition cells. An adult ape typically has 7,000.

Intuition cells are more numerous in your right brain. Your right frontal insula has 30 percent more than your left insula. Intuition cells appear to be designed to relay information rapidly from the salience network to other parts of the brain. They contain receptors for brain chemicals involved in social bonds, the expectation of reward under conditions of uncertainty, and for detecting danger, as well as for certain gut-based signaling molecules such as serotonin—all ingredients of intuition. When you think your luck is about to change while playing blackjack, these cells are active.

John Allman, a neuroscientist at Caltech and a leading expert on the VENs, says that when you meet someone, you create a mental model of how that person thinks and feels. You have initial, quick intuitions about the person—calling on your database of gut feelings, stereotypes, and subliminal perceptions—which are followed seconds, hours, or years later by slower, more reasoned judgments. We now know that when you make fast decisions, your frontal insula and anterior cingulate are active. These areas are also active when you experience pain, fear, nausea, or many social emotions. When you think something is funny, these same cells fire up, probably to recalibrate your intuitive judgments in changing situations. Humor serves to resolve uncertainty, relieve tension, engender trust, and promote social bonds.

It is believed that the rapid communication system involving the VENs may have evolved in mammals living in complex social organizations, enabling them to rapidly respond and adjust to quickly changing social situations through gut-based decision making. Because of their proposed role in social behavior, intuition, and empathy, it has been suggested that VEN abnormalities may contribute to the pathophysiology of autism spectrum disorders, including the compromised ability of these patients to empathize and interact socially. Although there's currently no direct scientific evidence to support this speculation, it's conceivable that the development of the VEN system in the brain is related to altered composition and function of the gut microbiota during the first few years in life, including the signals they send to the brain. Altered gut-brain communications have long been implicated in some forms of autism, and recent experiments using a mouse model of autism have identified altered gut microbe-to-brain signaling as a possible mechanism underlying these animals' autism-like behaviors.

DO ANIMALS HAVE GUT FEELINGS?

As humans, we take for granted our social emotions such as embarrassment, guilt, shame, and pride, and assume that animals, especially those we live with, must share the same feelings. Dog lovers swear that their canine companions experience emotions like shame, jealousy, anger, and affection in the same way we do.

However, if we go strictly by the anatomy of the brain, animals do not have the capacity to experience these emotions; their brains just aren't wired that way. The self-awareness of emotion conferred on humans by the anterior insula and its interactions with other cortical brain regions, in particular the prefrontal cortex, is unique. Dogs do have insulas but their frontal aspects are rudimentary. Internally generated sensations, including those from the gut, are integrated in the base of their brains and in subcortical emotional centers, rather than in the frontal insula. Dogs and other pets are clearly emotional but not self-aware, so no matter how human their emotional expressions appear, they are not in the same league with you, not matter how hard this is to accept.

Building Your Personal Google

Imagine that our memories of emotional moments are stored in our brains as tiny YouTube video clips. These videos contain not only the visuals of any given moment, but also the associated emotional, physical, attentional, and motivational components. We rarely remember the dates or specific circumstances of such events. Billions of these clips, or "somatic markers," are held in the biological equivalent of miniaturized servers in our brain and "annotated" (linked) with motivational states: a negative marker is associated with an unpleasant feeling and with the motivational drive of avoidance, whereas a positive marker is associated with a feeling of well-being and a motivational behavior to seek it out.

When we make a decision based on our gut feelings, the brain accesses the vast video library of emotional moments in our brains, like a Google search. In other words, you don't have to go through the time-consuming process of consciously considering all the possible positive and negative consequences of every particular decision you make. When faced with the need for action, your brain predicts how a given response will make you feel, based on its emotional memories of what took place when you were confronted with other, similar situations throughout your life. This probabilistic process then guides you away from responses that are likely to make you feel bad—

that is, anxious, pained, sick, sad, and so on—and toward responses that are linked to memories of feeling comfortable, happy, cared for, etc. Besides allowing you to make decisions more quickly, this mechanism lets you benefit from the past lessons without the psychological burden of reliving them. If you were to constantly revisit and relive your painful and unpleasant experiences, you'd go insane.

WOMEN'S INTUITION

In my experience with patients, many women seem to be better at listening to their gut feelings and making intuitive decisions than men are. The growing interest in identifying sex-related differences in emotional processing and in the prevalence of chronic pain conditions led to a series of studies funded by the National Institutes of Health aimed at identifying sex-related differences in brain responses to painful and emotional stimuli.

For a variety of political and convenience reasons, the study of such biological differences between women and men has been largely neglected, as it is automatically assumed that the female brain responds to such stimuli, as well as to medications, in the same way as the male brain. However, research by our group and others suggests that women tend to show greater sensitivity to the brain's salience and emotional arousal systems attuned to physical feelings like abdominal pain and emotional feelings like sadness or fear, than men do. One explanation of these differences may have to do with the fact that women store memories of physiologically painful or uncomfortable states such as menstruation, pregnancy, and childbirth. When expecting a potentially

painful experience, the female brain has a more extensive somatic marker library to go by, and its salience
system may have greater input from such memories
than the male system.

Are Decisions Based on Our Gut Feelings Always Right?

If what we know or reasonably suspect about gut feelings is
true, then shouldn't gut-feeling-based decisions be the best decisions?

Yes and no. While gut feelings are more informed by our
own experiences and learned knowledge than we may have
ever considered, they are also easily corrupted by a variety of
outside influences, including traumatic experiences, mood disorders, and advertising messages.

For example, TV programming is full of commercials targeted directly at your gut feelings, whether the aim is to moti-
vate you to eat a hamburger, go on a diet, or take a medication.
These cleverly designed commercials capture your attention by
presenting images, including an implicit promise of reward,
that are embedded smoothly and effortlessly into your stored
library of gut feelings and experiences.

Take, for example, the advertising slogan for a brand of peanut butter that says, "Choosy moms choose Jif." Being choosy
with regard to your children's health is a gut feeling that most
parents have; it's laudable. Advertisers and other influences
can hijack such basic gut feelings by taking advantage of the
fact that you're busy. You may consolidate and simplify information. Your gut-based desire to "be choosy when feeding your
children" combines with the slogan "choosy moms choose

Jif" in your brain to form the imperative "choose Jif," which is then mistaken for a gut feeling. So the question becomes not whether you can trust your gut feelings, but how you can learn to accurately identify what your true gut feelings are. Although the circuitry for making instantaneous gut-based, intuitive decisions evolved to enable you to live and navigate in complex societies, your challenge today is to use your gut to understand what is meaningful to you.

Our ability to make gut-feeling-based predictions and decisions is a by-product of evolution; in a dangerous world filled with life-threatening situations, a systemic bias toward assuming a high likelihood of bad outcomes can provide a significant survival advantage. Today, however, such a system has become maladaptive in most parts of the developed world, where life-threatening physical threats have largely been replaced by daily psychological stressors—the result being that our negatively biased gut-based decisions now result primarily in unhappiness and negative health outcomes.

A good example of this is the story of Frank. He had to force himself to go to lunch meetings with his clients, because his brain's predictions regarding what would happen in an unfamiliar restaurant created so much anxiety and related gastrointestinal symptoms that he was unable to focus on the meeting. This phenomenon is known as catastrophizing, which simply means that your brain makes the (wrong) gut-feeling-based prediction that the worst possible outcome (in this case, severe digestive symptoms) will occur. The instant Frank found out about a new appointment, his intuitive, negatively biased prediction of future events in the restaurant kicked in, preventing him from rationally assessing the situation. Catastrophizing is also a common trait in patients suffering from depression or chronic pain, whose attention is narrowed to only negative stimuli. Some people with these conditions have completely lost the ability to make gut-feeling-based decisions that are good for their well-being.

HOW WE DECIDE

When it comes to buying a bottle of wine, there are three types of strategies, depending on your decision-making strategy.

First are the linear, rational types who base their decision on what they have learned in a wine-tasting class (the best years for that particular varietal, the amount of sugar added, the age, and so on) or from reading the newsletter published by a famous wine master. Gut sensation experts, on the other hand, make their decisions based on a natural or trained ability to detect an astonishing number of different flavors and aromas (ranging from chocolate to raspberry to cinnamon) when smelling and tasting a particular wine. Finally, there are the intuitive types, the gut feeling experts, who over their lifetime have accumulated a vast library of emotional memories related to wine consumption. These memories may include enjoyable moments experienced in a small town in Tuscany or Provence, or drinking a simple bottle of red wine with delicious food in the company of good friends. Memories may also include the fragrance of the surrounding lavender fields and the thunderstorm that drove everybody from the outdoor restaurant inside. The gut feelings generated and stored during these pleasant experiences contain not only the actual taste of the wine (the gut sensation), but also the context (beautiful scenery) and the feeling state (being relaxed, happy, or in love).

When you watch the three types making a decision about which wine to buy, the rational type will do searches on the Internet and carefully, logically weigh the price, year, and other learned information about the wine. The sensory experts may go to a wine-tasting room to discover the ultimate blend of flavors and aromas. Meanwhile, the intuitive type will be influenced primarily by the memories they may have about the particular part of the world where the wine originated, or about the occasion at which they shared the wine in good company.

Accessing Your Gut Feelings Through Dreams

If we were able to watch a gut-feeling-based documentary of our lives, composed of all these individual clips spliced together, we would presumably witness a fascinating, highly personal biopic, played out in vivid colors.

But short of such a fantasy, how might we catch a glimpse of the video library in our minds? Watching our own emotional biopic during waking hours, when we're busy dealing with the challenging world around us, would be incredibly distracting. A much more plausible time to view such a movie would be at night, when we are not distracted by work, family, or friends, and when our body is temporarily offline and won't move during even the scariest scenes. And in fact, that's exactly when showtime occurs for this cinema of the emotions—when we are asleep, or, more specifically, when we are absorbed in our dreams.

The experience of dreaming can often seem as if we are

actually watching a movie, and anybody who is able to remember his or her dreams will agree that the human brain is a remarkable film director. It is generally assumed that the most vivid dreams occur during the period of sleep called rapid eye movement (REM) sleep. During REM sleep, your breathing becomes more rapid, irregular, and shallow, your eyes jerk rapidly in various directions, and your brain becomes extremely active. Movies of particular personal relevance play more frequently, and appear in more colorful and emotional formats.

Brain imaging studies in sleeping subjects demonstrated that the brain regions activated during REM sleep include the familiar salience network regions of the insula and cingulate cortex, along with several emotion-generating regions—including the amygdala, and regions involved in memory, such as the hippocampus and the orbitofrontal cortex—as well as the brain region essential for experiencing the images, the visual cortex. At the same time, brain areas involved in cognitive control and conscious awareness, including the prefrontal and parietal cortexes, and regions controlling voluntary movement are turned off. You are paralyzed. This way, we can experience an uncensored version of our film without worrying that we'll fall out of bed when we feel like running away or punching someone in the face. You cannot enact your dreams, unless you have a rare sleep disorder.

Interestingly, while our body movements are turned off, the brain-gut-microbiota axis is more active during sleep than at any other time. The migrating motor complex—the powerful contractions and bursts of gastrointestinal secretions, discussed in Chapter 2, that pass through our intestines every ninety minutes when there is no food in our gastrointestinal tract—are fully activated during sleep, and dramatically change the environment for our gut microbes (and presumably their metabolic activity) during this period. Based on what we know today, it is likely that these contractile waves are also associated with release of the many signaling molecules in the gut and with transmission of this information to the brain, via the many gut-to-brain communication channels. Even though no scientific studies have been done to prove this point, I wouldn't be surprised if such bursts of intense gut- and microbe-to-brain signaling, with all the neuroactive substances being released during this process, play a role in the affective coloring of our dreams.

Why is dreaming significant? One proposed theory is that dreaming during REM sleep helps to integrate and consolidate various aspects of our emotional memories. As I'll discuss later, dream analysis is one way to get in touch with and learn to trust your gut feelings. While there are many other hypotheses about the role and importance of dreams, the idea that one of its functions is to consolidate the emotional memories in the form of gut feelings that we accumulated during the day fits much of the scientific data that has been gathered in this field. Some intriguing recent findings, for example, suggest that the gut-brain axis, possibly including signals from the microbiota, plays an important role in the modulation of REM sleep and dream states. So the next time you have a late meal just before going to bed, or get up in the middle of the night to forage in your refrigerator, you might think about the unintended effect this may have on your nighttime movie showing, and the updating of your internal database!

A quarter-century ago, at a time when I was overwhelmed by decisions I had to make about my own life's direction, I was fortunate to have gone through Jungian psychoanalysis for several years. Carl Gustav Jung was a famous psychiatrist at the Burghölzli psychiatric hospital in Zurich, Switzerland, and a contemporary of Sigmund Freud. He was the founder of analytical psychology, an elaborate conceptualization of psychology that includes such key concepts as a shared (collective) unconscious; universal, inborn patterns of unconscious images (so-called archetypes) that guide our behavior; and the concept of individuation, a psychological process of integrating opposite psychological tendencies, like introversion and extroversion. Jung saw dream analysis as the key strategy to get access to our unconscious. Today I speculate that the latter process has a lot to do with getting in touch with, and learning to trust, your gut feelings.

While I had always been fascinated by Jung's writings about dream analyses, I wasn't quite ready for the recurrent weekly questions from my therapist regarding the dreams I'd had since our last appointment. While I had begun my therapy looking for practical help on making the most *rational* decisions about my future, my therapist consistently redirected me to look inside myself and find the answers from my dreams.

There were weeks when I was terrified, driving to my weekly appointment without a single dream written down in my journal, facing a session where there would be nothing to talk about. Over a matter of months, however, the dreams I was able to remember steadily increased in their frequency, detail, and intensity. I was amazed at the beauty, story lines, and complexity of the "inner movies" that I was watching every night. The most elaborate of these dreams, associated with the strongest feelings, turned out to be the ones with the greatest personal meaning. The combination of writing down my dreams every morning and then reflecting on them, with or without my therapist, gradually brought me to a point where I was able to connect with my internal database of emotional memories, and began trusting my inner wisdom reflected in these dreams more and more in making important decisions, rather than relying on the advice of friends and colleagues.

But dream analysis is not the only way to get in touch with your gut feelings. There are other ways of training yourself to listen to your gut feelings that are less cumbersome and expensive than Jungian psychoanalysis. Ericksonian hypnosis is one. Milton Erickson, a famous hypnotherapist, was a master at putting his patients into a trance by directing his elaborate, hypnosis-inducing stories alternatively to the conscious, rational (left) side of the brain and to the wise, all-knowing unconscious (right) side of the brain. Over the course of the hypnotic induction, the subject would come to trust the unconscious side more and more, while letting go of any attempt to control things through rational, linear thought mechanisms. Not only is hypnosis a highly effective way of rapidly switching the brain from an external attentional focus to an introspective mode, thereby inducing a trance, but repeated sessions of Ericksonian hypnosis also change the way patients make important decisions when they are not in a trance state. Over time, many of Erickson's regular subjects increasingly learned to trust this inner wisdom and make their decisions accordingly.

The Bottom Line

We use the expression "gut feeling" frequently in our daily conversations, without realizing that a tremendous amount of cumulative scientific evidence provides the biological underpinnings for this term. The quality, accuracy, and underlying biases of this gut-brain dialogue vary between different individuals. Some gut sensations are recorded with high fidelity and are replayed in a subliminal way: Even though they rarely reach our consciousness, such movies, like dreams, are likely to play an important role in our background feeling states. In addition, certain individuals seem to be more sensitive and aware of all signals coming from the gut. They may view themselves as always having had a "sensitive stomach" or may have been told by their mothers that they were colicky babies. Some learn to live with this hypersensitivity and accept it as part of their personality. They will tell you that they are more sensitive to food and medications and will feel butterflies in their stomach when anxious. Others in this group develop common gastrointestinal disorders such as IBS, as their brain, flooded by a constant stream of aberrant signals from the gut, generates inappropriate gut reactions based on the signals received.

By getting in touch with our gut feelings, understanding the role that our personal collection of gut-based memories plays in our intuitive decision making, and keeping in mind that whatever we do to influence the activities of our gut microbes—through our diet or medication intake—may also influence our emotions and predictions about the future, we can fully tap into the vast potential of the gut-microbiota-brain axis.

It seems strange that given the crucial importance of gut-based decision making, there is no formal mechanism in place to train and optimize this remarkable ability. We certainly don't learn about it in school, and many parents don't tell their children to listen to their gut, instead stressing the importance of thinking things through logically (which, of course, is also a valuable skill for impulsive adolescents to practice). The ultimate dogma of modern society is to make rational decisions based on the assumption that the world is linear and predictable, and that if you have enough information about the world, you can make the best decisions. I strongly believe that once we gain a better understanding of the biological underpinnings of intuitive decision making and accept it as a worthwhile goal to invest our mental energies in improving these skills, there is a range of strategies we can embark on to improve our ability and inclination for gut-feeling-based decision making later in life.

||||||||||||||||||||||||||||||||||

PART 3

HOW TO

OPTIMIZE

BRAIN-GUT

HEALTH

CHAPTER

8

THE ROLE OF FOOD: LESSONS FROM HUNTER- GATHERERS

|||||||||||||||||||||||||||||||||||||||||||||||||||||||||||||||||||||||||||||||||||||||||||||||||||||||||||||||||||||||||||||||

A ll around the world, food is central to the human social experience. We sit around the holiday table and listen and laugh as family members swap stories. We meet new friends over dinner, and sometimes they become more than friends. We hold breakfast meetings, award luncheons, and potluck dinners. As often as not, the affairs of human life involve breaking bread together.

Yet as the pace of modern life has accelerated, our eating habits have changed. We've moved from sit-down meals with the family to fast-food burgers to frozen entrees to processed snacks to meals that can be ordered at the touch of a button. Through those decades in the United States, many of us were haunted by the feeling that something as central to our existence as our diet was becoming profoundly *un*natural. The enduring and appealing backlash to that trend, embodied in natural food restaurants, farmer's markets, and the slow-food movement, reveals a deeper yearning to find what we lost in all that modernization—to uncover what was good and natural and healthy about our sustenance.

How can we recover what we've lost? We can start by looking at the science. Over millions of years, our digestive systems, gut microbes, and brains evolved together, honing our instinctive ability to locate, harvest, and prepare food that is good for us and to avoid unhealthy food. And for almost all of that time, we obtained our food by hunting and gathering. Could the diet of the earliest hunter-gatherers guide us in the right direction?

At the same time, we have to remember that humans can thrive on a tremendously diverse array of diets. From the handpicked tubers, berries, and fruits of Tanzania's hunter-gatherers to the seals, whales, and narwhals of the meat-loving Inuit, traditional cultures thrived for generations on the most diverse of fare. Agrarian farmers, in contrast, relied on wheat, corn, rice, and other staple grains, as well as vegetables, with some meat, and perhaps milk, cheese, and yogurt from domesticated animals. Because of our digestive versatility, people have managed to find sustenance in a tremendous variety of climate conditions and environments.

Part of the credit for that feat goes to our own amazing GI tract and its connection with the computing power of our nervous system. Millions of years of evolution have perfected the gut to sense, recognize, and encode everything we eat and drink into patterns of hormones and nerve impulses sent to regulatory centers in the brain. But as we have learned, a large part of the credit also goes to our gut microbiota, which take care of the variable fraction of our food that cannot be absorbed in the small intestine. Taken collectively, human gut microbiota are incredibly diverse and marvelously adaptable, and over millions of years of evolution they have become an indispensable link in our digestive process.

In North America today, it's hard to get away from an unnatural diet, one that's full of sweeteners, emulsifiers, flavorings, and colorings, with extra fat, added sugar, and vital gluten, and loaded with calories. Since the food we eat influences the activity of our microbiota, what exactly would our microbiota look like if we ate the diet our bodies evolved with? What does our ancestral microbiome tell us? Can we ever even know what it was?

In fact, we can. And learning more about our true ancestral diet may even provide some answers to the never-ending debate over which diet is best for our bodies and minds: the high-fat/high-protein, low-carb variety, the high-fruit and -vegetable omnivore diet, the extremes of the vegan diet, or the tasty compromise of the Mediterranean diet. And in so doing, we can get a glimpse to a time when our brains, guts, and gut microbes were living in harmony—a glimpse of the diet we have evolved to eat.

One way to do this is by studying people who still follow a prehistoric lifestyle, whose diet is not much different from the diet our bodies evolved to eat over tens of thousands of years. I'm talking about the world's remaining primitive agrarians or hunter-gatherers—rural Malawians and the Yanomami.

Dietary Lessons from the Yanomami

Forty years ago, I had a fascinating personal experience that gave me a firsthand look at the Yanomami and their eating habits. It involved a journey that took me thousands of miles into the Venezuelan jungle, to a part of the Amazon rain forest that is the homeland of a primal people living around the headwaters of the Orinoco River.

My rain forest experience was brought back to me in unexpected fashion in 2013, when I attended a major scientific conference on the gut microbiome in Bethesda, Maryland. The conference was titled "Human Microbiome Science: Vision for the Future." One of the conference presenters was ecologist and microbiologist Maria Gloria Dominguez-Bello, an internationally renowned scientist who has authored landmark papers on how the mode of delivery influences the gut microbiota of newborn babies. She was also part of a team of investigators that published a comparison of the gut microbial composition among different groups, including Amerindians (a group of indigenous people found in South America) and people living in North American cities.

When I saw her first slides of the indigenous people living along the Orinoco River, I couldn't believe my eyes: the images of these short, beautiful people, with their distinctive features and unique monklike hairstyles, immediately brought back memories from 1972, when I was fortunate to be invited by a documentary filmmaker to serve as a camera assistant in a film expedition to the Yanomami. I was in my first year of college, and it didn't take much for me to decide to take a semester off and embark on this unique adventure.

Since I didn't know much about anthropology or medicine at the time—not to mention the gut microbiota, which hadn't even been discovered in their full magnitude—my main motivation for going on this expedition was a mix of pure adventure-seeking and fascination at being part of a documentary film production. However, preparing for the expedition, I also learned about one unique aspect of the Yanomami's eating habits: the complete lack of salt as a food additive. Several studies have linked low sodium consumption by the Yanomami with a virtual absence of high blood pressure and its medical complications. But now, after decades of clinical practice and research into the complex dialogue between the brain, gut, and microbiome, I realized that there were much more intriguing things about the Yanomami diet, which not only influence their health but possibly also their minds and behaviors.

I bring up this personal story because the Yanomami are one of a handful of people in the world who have continued to follow the prehistoric lifestyle that our ancestors lived tens of thousands of years ago. Studying their eating habits and their gut microbiomes gives us a window back in time, to the period when humans and microbes first started their symbiotic lives together. This research can give us clues about how our gut microbes evolved, and the consequences this may have for our well-being today.

Along with the other two members of our film team, I lived in a Yanomami village for two months. I had a chance to observe and experience their daily lives, including how they collected, prepared, and consumed their food. I saw and tasted what they ate on a daily basis and also experienced their unique range of emotional behaviors, ranging from the affectionate interactions of fathers with their newborns, to the violent, ritualistic fistfights that took place during a major celebration, to their preparations to go to war against another village.

Following an initial prolonged and noisy ritual of familiarization, during which the entire village touched our heads, faces, chests, and arms, and after each of us was assigned a hammock, the village people pretty much ignored the filmmakers living in their midst—except for the children, who wanted to touch and play with everything we had in our backpacks, including our cameras. This gave us a unique opportunity to watch and film their daily routines and observe their behaviors, particularly their activities related to foraging and harvesting.

Yanomamis have a strict division of labor related to foraging: the men go hunting for birds, monkeys, deer, wild pigs, and tapirs (all wild animals with minimal body fat), which can take up to 60 percent of their time. We would often see several men leaving the shabono with bow and arrow in the early morning hours and returning later in the day with their prey. The meat from these animals is roasted or baked; because they don't use any oils or animal fats, nothing is fried. The women would hang the prepared meat pieces on a pole within the family area, including monkey heads and pieces of snakes, frogs, and birds, together with bushels of platanos, a form of banana.

It was a common sight to see family members nibbling on these stored food supplies throughout the day, and I was often invited to join in during the snacks. Despite the abundance of wild animals in the forest, animal products account for only a small percentage of the Yanomami's food supply. Furthermore, our guide informed us that the Yanomamis never eat their domestic animals, which are mainly kept as pets, or bird eggs, which they only use for spiritual purposes and ceremonies. The women are involved in horticulture, growing a form of sweet potato as well as platanos and tobacco. We followed and filmed them on their long foraging trips into the forest to collect grubs, termites, frogs, honey, and seedlings. Both men and women shared the activity of catching fish out of the pristine water of the rivers. Procuring their food involves extensive physical exercise, including prolonged walking and running through the rain forest. Keeping up with their pace in this hot and humid environment was not an easy task.

The Yanomami families depend on the enormous diversity of the forest for survival, and the high diversity of their environment is reflected in the diversity of their gut microbiomes. In addition to their staple diet of fruit and vegetables, they also employ a large number of plant products for other purposes, including various plant-derived poisons that are used to make deadly arrowheads for fishing and hunting, and hundreds of different plants, berries, and seeds that are consumed for dietary, medicinal, and hallucinogenic purposes. The Yanomamis also employ the principle of fermentation in their food preparation, providing them with a natural supply of microorganisms. We witnessed how a group of people smashed a large amount of platanos into a puree inside of a dugout canoe until natural fermentation turned the slurry into an alcoholic beverage, which the men then consumed in large quantities, with noticeable consequences for their behavior. Perhaps the Yanomami, through centuries of trial and error, had learned something about how compounds from both food and medicinal plants provide specific signals, triggering effects on both our brain and our gut.

Overall, the Yanomamis' diet was rich in plant foods, supplemented with occasional bits of meat. But unlike the processed and fat-enriched beef and pork products that make up the bulk of our North American meat supply, the meat the Yanomamis ate came from animals that were wild, lean, and healthy. The Yanomami live a long way from the nutrition gurus who fill today's bookshelves and airwaves, but their diet—rich in vegetables, fruit, and occasional fish and lean meat, with no additives or preservatives at all—is in line with Michael Pollan's well-known advice from *The Omnivore's Dilemma*: "Eat food, not too much, mostly plants."

I am in no way suggesting that you should become a hunter-gatherer; I do not believe that we should all eat a Paleolithic diet for optimal health. These indigenous people show stunted growth (which is adaptive for their lives as hunter-gatherers in the forest), their life expectancy doesn't even come close to ours, and they have a high rate of mortality from wars and injuries. At the same time, observing their lifestyle does provide a unique opportunity to learn about the intertwined roles of diet and the gut microbiome in promoting good human health.

Is the North American Diet Bad for Your Gut Microbes?

Can a lean diet, rich in a variety of plant foods with a small proportion of meat, help support the health of your gut microbiota? And has our modern North American diet altered human gut microbiota for the worse? Only in the last few years have scientists begun to uncover some answers.

A few years ago, Tanya Yatsunenko, Maria Gloria Dominguez-Bello, and a team of prominent microbiome experts under the leadership of Jeffrey Gordon from Washington University assessed the gut microbial composition of the Guahibos, an indigenous Amazonian tribe living in the same region as the Yanomamis; rural people from an agrarian village in the southern African nation of Malawi; and North American city dwellers. The researchers used modern methods known as metagenomics: they isolated all the gut microbes from fecal samples, purified their genetic material (DNA), then used an automated analysis technique to identify all the bacterial genes. Using this technique, they found that gut microbiota from the South American Indians and the rural Malawians were composed of a similar mix of microbes, but a mix that's very different from that of North Americans. At first glance, these findings wouldn't be too surprising, given the vastly different lifestyles and eating habits of us and these primal people living in very different geographic and cultural settings.

The Malawians and Amerindians are genetically different and live in very different tropical environments—the Amazonian rain forest, which provides a fairly constant climate year-round, versus the arid savanna of Malawi, which has marked wet and dry seasons—so what accounts for the similarity? It turns out that in both of these traditional societies, people consume a similar diet with a large variety of plant-based foods as well as occasional lean meat from animals they've hunted themselves.

In fact, the Malawians and Amerindians had a similar pattern of microbes in their gut that make up a telltale signature for humans adhering to a diet high in plant and low in animal products, a reduced ratio of the bacterial phyla of Firmicutes to Bacteroidetes, and, within the Bacteroidetes group, an increased ratio of the groups Prevotella and Bacteroides. Other studies comparing children from rural areas of the West African country of Burkina Faso to children from Florence, Italy, or Hazda hunter-gatherers from Tanzania's Eastern Rift Valley to adults from Bologna, Italy, have confirmed these essential findings.

As the studies in hunter-gatherer populations mentioned above were all performed at a single time point, they didn't allow us to account for the known seasonal variations in dietary intake in the Hazdas or Malawians, and the possible effect on gut microbial composition and function. However, a recent study by Justin Sonnenburg's group at Stanford University, published in the journal *Science*, shed light on this important question. As Sonnenburg points out, food acquisition consumes a major part of the Hazda's activities, and the pattern of these activities are subject to two distinct seasons: the wet season between November and April, and the dry season between May and October. While the consumption of fiber-rich tuber and of the fruit of the baobab treat is more or less constant throughout the year, the consumption of meat greatly increases during the dry season which is more conducive to hunting. In contrast, the Hazdas indulge in sugary berries and honey during the wet season. The most fascinating aspect of their study was the observation that the gut microbial composition and function changed in synchrony with the dominant diet: Microbial diversity decreased during the dry season with the consumption of meat to a level similar to that seen in Western populations, but increased significantly during the wet season when fruit and vegetable consumption increased. The very microbial species that were seasonally volatile in the Hazdas are the ones that appear to be permanently lost in Western populations. When the authors compared their data collected from eighteen populations from sixteen countries with varying lifestyles, they realized that the gut microbial community structure was closely related to modernization with the organisms fluctuating seasonally in the Hazda, being the same ones that differentiated industrialized from traditional populations.

Most worrisome about the findings from a growing number of such studies is the fact that they consistently show that people living on the typical North American diet had lost up to one-third of their microbial diversity compared to individuals living a prehistoric lifestyle. And here's an equally concerning thought: this dramatic change in our gut-based ecosystem is directly comparable to the estimated 30 percent loss of biodiversity that our planet has experienced since 1970—much of which has occurred in the Amazonian rain forest, the habitat of the Yanomami. Unfortunately, this decrease in biodiversity around the world is not limited to plants and animals living in subtropical rain forests, and ecologists have developed elegant mathematical models to characterize its effect on various ecosystems. Decreased biodiversity affects the marine life living on the coral reefs, and the honeybees and monarch butterflies in North America. Can we use the same insights ecologists have gained from studying the decline of the ecosystems around us to understand the consequences of the declining biodiversity inside our guts? Just as greater diversity in natural systems provides resilience against diseases, greater diversity and richness in a host's microbial species and their metabolites is associated with greater resilience in the face of infections, antibiotics, variable nutrient supply, carcinogenic chemicals, and chronic stress.

Not everyone in North America follows the typical regional diet, of course. Similar to societies that subsist on agrarian and prehistoric diets, traditional Asian or European diets and vegetarians have lower intakes of saturated fat and cholesterol and higher intakes of fruits, vegetables, whole grains, nuts, soy products, fiber, and phytochemicals (chemical substances that occur naturally in plants). And many populations around the world follow a pattern of seasonal variation of their food intake, analogous to the example of the Hazdas. However, there is substantial scientific evidence showing significant health benefits from eating diets of this type that are high in plant food and low in animal-derived components, especially fat. For example, many studies have demonstrated that people who eat vegetarian or vegan diets have a reduced prevalence of obesity, metabolic syndrome, coronary vascular disease, hypertension, and stroke, as well as a reduced risk of cancer. Unfortunately, there's very little evidence to date indicating that such diets also have direct benefits for brain health—which is to say, benefits that aren't simply a reflection of better physical health.

As impressive as the differences in gut microbial abundance and diversity were in the adult subjects in the Yatsunenko study, investigators found that differences in gut microbiomes between the South American Indian and African groups and the North American city dwellers were not necessarily dependent on the lifestyle of the adult subjects, but they were already apparent during the first three years of life and persisted into adulthood. What might be responsible for these gut microbial differences so early in life, before infants have been exposed to the different diets of the adults?

Where It All Begins

Food plays a key part in the health of our gut, our brain, and in the interaction of the two vital organs, and this close relationship starts the moment we are born. While we all want to optimize our health as adults, the findings of the Yatsunenko study remind us that we must not forget that some of the most consequential influences of food on the gut microbiome start long before we can make our own decisions about what we eat and which probiotics we choose. These early food-related influences on our gut microbiome set the foundation for our adult gut microbial diversity and resilience against disease, and errors in this process in this early programming can increase our risk for a range of health problems, ranging from obesity to IBS. In addition to the initial shaping of a baby's gut microbiome during birth, the food the child receives from her mother plays a crucial role in this process. A study by microbiologist Ruth Ley of Cornell University and her team highlighted this important influence of early diet on the gut microbiota of a healthy baby boy, analyzed at sixty time points from birth to age two and a half.

The boy was breastfed exclusively for his first four and a half months. At first, Ley and her colleagues found, the infant's microbiome was rich in species that facilitate the digestion of milk carbohydrates, primarily bifidobacteria and some lactobacilli. This was not surprising. But before he had consumed any formula or a bite of solid food, gut microbes such as Prevotella appeared that could metabolize complex carbohydrates from plants. This meant that the baby's gut microbiota were prepared for solid food before the baby had ever eaten any.

The baby's mother continued to breastfeed him until he was nine months old, and the parents gradually phased in baby foods like rice cereal and peas, then table foods. Once the baby was switched to solid food, the microbiota switched again to microbes that ferment plant carbohydrates.

In the early months of the baby's life, relatively few species lived in the gut, and events such as a fever, introduction of peas to his diet, or antibiotic treatment for an ear infection caused the child's microbial communities to fluctuate dramatically. But the diversity climbed by the month, and by the time the boy was two and a half years old, his gut microbiome had stabilized and come to resemble that of an adult.

From this and other studies, it's now clear that those first two and a half to three years shape our gut microbiome for a lifetime. It's as if a child's body were staffing a symphony orchestra, with each species of gut bacteria playing a single instrument. At first players try out. Some are hired and some are not, but many seats remain empty. By age two and a half, however, the orchestra is fully staffed, and the majority of players have their jobs for life. Depending on the circumstances, and the food supply, this orchestra is able to play a repertoire of different tunes.

The Crucial Role of Diet in Shaping a Baby's Gut-Brain Dialogue

In recent years, as we've learned more about the connections between brain, gut, and microbiome, I've thought back occasionally to the Yanomami teenager who had given birth to a baby in the Venezuelan jungle, and whom I watched interacting with the newborn for several weeks. I regularly saw the young mother joining the other women in the village to collect food items, while carrying her baby with help of a shoulder strap over her chest and belly, breastfeeding her throughout the day.

The baby seemed perfectly healthy, and based on what I witnessed and what investigators have since learned, the baby's gut—and its gut microbiota—were off to a healthy start, showing high abundance and diversity of microorganisms. From birth onward, this girl was exposed not only to the vast microbial diversity of her natural environment, but also to the unique components of the food she received from her mother.

We know today that it's the infant's food supply, in particular breast milk, which helps her gut fill with the initial healthy mix of microbes. Keep in mind that the composition of breast milk is crucially dependent on the diet the mother consumes. Recent studies have shown that the composition of the nursing mother's diet has a major influence on the baby's risk for metabolic disease and obesity later on in life, and much of this is mediated by the early programming of the baby's gut microbiota. While mothers have always known that breast milk is the optimal food for their infants, recent gut microbiome science has revealed unexpected mechanisms by which this health benefit is mediated. Besides all the nutrients essential for the child's development, breast milk contains prebiotics—compounds with the ability to feed particular groups of gut microbes. Specifically it contains oligosaccharides—complex carbohydrates made of three to ten linked sugar molecules—that are essential in shaping the baby's gut microbiota by selectively promoting the growth of beneficial bacteria. These carbohydrates, called human milk oligosaccharides, or HMOs, form the third-largest component of human breast milk, and more than 150 distinct HMO molecules have been identified.

What's fascinating about HMOs is that women's bodies make them despite the fact that they are indigestible by the human gut. These molecules resist the acidity in an infant's stomach as well as digestion by pancreatic and small intestinal enzymes, reaching the end of the small intestine and colon (where the great majority of our gut microbes live) in an intact form. Once they reach their target, they nourish beneficial microbiota, in particular *Bifidobacterium* species that are able to partially break them down into short-chain fatty acids and other metabolites. These breakdown products create an environment favoring the growth of good microbes over potential pathogens. This helps explain the fact that infants who are not breastfed have fewer bifidobacteria in their stool than formula-fed infants. As David Mills of the University of California, Davis, who is one of the world's experts on the components of human milk, points out, HMOs are the only food that has evolved strictly for the purpose of feeding the infant's microbiota. Clearly, evolution has designed these molecules specifically to help program the baby's gut microbiota, while at the same time providing protection against pathogenic bacteria. One way they accomplish this is by favoring the dominance of *Bifidobacterium infantis* (microbes that are experts in digesting them), thereby preventing the growth of potentially harmful bacteria as they compete for a limited nutrient supply. In addition, HMOs have direct antimicrobial effects against such pathogens, which is reflected in a reduction of microbial infections affecting the infant. Thus HMOs are essential to the development of a healthy infant microbiome, and for the temporary protection against intestinal infections, at a time when the infant's microbiome has a low diversity (made up of a limited number of microbial groups and species) and is not ready yet to defend effectively against infections.

Evolution has come up with a beautiful seamless transition

of the nearly microbe-free fetus into a world teeming with microorganisms, by first using the unique microbial environment of the mother's vagina to inoculate the sterile gut of the newborn, then promoting the growth of these same microbes in the gut of the infant with specific molecules contained in human breast milk long enough for the growing infant to develop its own unique microbial composition.

During my two months with the Yanomami, I saw mothers breastfeeding not just infants, but also toddlers. In fact, they breastfeed for three full years while adding platanos to this early diet after the first year, as do many other traditional hunter-gatherer societies. During that period, a child's gut microbiome is not the only thing that is taking shape—her brain is as well. Brain development continues through adolescence, but the first few years of life are especially critical. Can breastfeeding change the gut-microbiota-brain conversation to promote healthy development of critical brain circuits and systems?

Long-term studies of breastfed infants suggest that it can. Several longitudinal studies have followed such infants until they grew up, with the scientists measuring their cognitive and intellectual abilities along the way. Such studies, in which researchers obtain measurements on subjects periodically over the years, offer a movie showing how a particular process develops; most important, they can reveal cause and effect. The longitudinal studies on breastfed infants have shown that the longer an infant is breastfed, the larger his brain is, a trait associated with improved cognitive development.

Breastfeeding can even enhance a baby's emotional and social development. In recent work from a team of investigators at the Max Planck Institute for Human Cognitive and Brain Sciences in Leipzig, Germany, investigators tested eight-month-old infants who had been exclusively breastfed earlier in their lives, for their ability to recognize emotion from a person's body language, depicted by images of a person who was happy or showed expressions of fear. The results were dramatic: the infants who were breastfed longer responded more to happy body expressions than those who had been breastfed for a shorter period. Recognizing basic emotions like happiness or anger from facial expressions and body language gives babies a fundamental tool that's crucial to their emotional and social development.

How does breastfeeding specifically alter the brain regions responsible for learning these skills? The results of the German study suggest that it does so in part through the action of oxytocin. A variety of sensory stimuli cause oxytocin release in the brain: gentle touch, nursing a child, or certain gut sensations caused by nutrients. The hormone is released in the brains of both the nursing mother (where it stimulates the flow of milk) and her infant. Oxytocin promotes affiliation and bonding, suggesting that oxytocin release during nursing enhances mother-child bonding. In a follow-up study, it was reported that this positive effect of prolonged breastfeeding was dependent on the genetic makeup of the infants, as it was only seen in infants who had a particular genetic variation in the signaling system for oxytocin.

While fascinating by themselves, the studies on the relationship between breastfeeding and emotional reactivity didn't address the question of which aspect of the breastfeeding was responsible for the oxytocin release in the brain. "Breast feeding is much more than simply a meal at the breast," writes the lead author, Tobias Grossmann, and his colleagues. So was it the positive experiences of the infant associated with prolonged body contact that came with the breastfeeding, the oral stimulation (which stimulates oxytocin release in the mother), or the consumption of milk sugar (which can stimulate the release of opioid-like molecules in the brain)? Or was it some metabolite, such as the Valium-like amino acid GABA, which the infant's gut microbiota produced in response to the regular delivery of human milk oligosaccharides to the intestine, and which signaled the brain that all is good?

In the brain-imaging study our UCLA group did on adult female volunteers who ate probiotic-enriched yogurt regularly, probiotics affected the activity of some of the same emotional brain regions that were affected in the breastfed babies in Grossmann's study described above. And in very recent studies, we found that there is a correlation between the volume of certain brain regions and the general composition of the gut microbiota. Is it possible that this relationship between the brain and the gut microbes develops early in life, during the time when both brain architecture and gut microbial composition are still under development? Based on what we know today, the amount and duration of delivery of human milk oligosaccharides to the infant's metabolic machinery in the gut could play a crucial role in this process.

Can a New Diet Alter Your Gut Microbiota?

When your diet changes, it can fundamentally alter living conditions for your gut microbes. But there are trillions of them in your gut, and many can reproduce quickly. This means that—in theory at least—natural selection could act quickly, allowing the best-adapted bugs to thrive and others to lie low or die off entirely.

But that's not the only possibility. Existing gut microbes

could also adapt to the new conditions by altering their gene expression to activate newly essential functions and turn off others that they no longer need. To find out which of these two possibilities is correct, and how a major dietary shift would alter the mix of microbes in the gut, several research groups investigated whether differences in dietary habits among people living in industrialized societies are reflected in changes in their gut microbiota and the metabolites they produce. Peter Turnbaugh's group at Harvard University studied the acute effect of switching healthy individuals from their normal diet to either a plant-based diet (rich in grains, legumes, fruits, and vegetables) or an extreme animal-based, high-fat diet (composed of meats, eggs, and cheeses).

The short-term switching of individuals from their regular diet to either a plant- or an animal-based diet also changed their gut microbial composition. The changes were similar to earlier reports about microbiome differences between herbivore and carnivore animals, and about gut microbial differences between Westerners and people eating a prehistoric diet. Interestingly, the animal-based high-fat diet had a greater effect on people's baseline microbiota composition and prevalence of certain species than the plant-based diet did, suggesting that it represented a greater deviation from the subjects' default diet than the plant-based diet did. Those on the animal-based diet also showed increased abundance of microorganisms tolerant to bile acids (bile acids are required to absorb fat in the small intestine) and had decreased levels of bacteria that metabolize complex sugar molecules contained in plants. When subjects who had been living on a vegetarian diet before the study were switched to the animal-based diet, microorganisms that are highly prevalent in prehistoric and agrarian societies were reduced, confirming the importance of this genus for metabolizing plant carbohydrates.

In addition to these changes in microbial organization, microbial metabolic activity showed diet-related changes as well. As expected, compared to the plant-based diet and the baseline diet, the animal-based diet resulted in a significantly higher concentration of products from amino acid fermentation, and lower levels of metabolites resulting from carbohydrate fermentation (in particular, short-chain fatty acids).

As the study's authors pointed out, the ability of the gut microbiota to rapidly shift its composition and functional profiles may have been important to mankind's survival, since it allows adjustment to variations in climate- and season-related availability of animal and plant foods. In addition, it probably had an adaptive value during the evolution of humans from our earliest evolutionary ancestors to today's *Homo sapiens*. The ability to quickly adapt to readily available plant foods during times of limited availability of meat may have provided an alternative source of calories and nutrients. The findings also may explain why humans can adjust to rapidly changing therapeutic and fad diets (for example, gluten-free, Atkins, paleo, and vegan diets) without major side effects and apparently without dramatic changes in mood, affect, or stress responsiveness.

Given this evidence that our gut microbiota can rapidly adapt to extreme short-term dietary changes, in terms of both their composition and the metabolites they produce, we might expect to see clear differences between individuals in a Western urban environment who have chosen to consume plant-based diets (vegan and vegetarian) compared to their omnivore neighbors. Surprisingly, a study by Gary Wu and his group at the University of Pennsylvania did not confirm this speculation. The investigators did a detailed analysis of the gut microbiota and gut-microbe-derived metabolites in a group of omnivores and in individuals who had been on a vegan diet for at least six months. Contrary to earlier study results regarding individuals who were born in and have lived in different geographic regions of the world for all their lives, they found only a modest difference in the gut microbiota of Westerners who had chosen their diets to be either omnivores or vegan. They did observe differences in the gut microbe metabolites of the two groups as measured in their blood and urine, however, largely reflecting the vegans' lower intake of protein and fat and higher intake of carbohydrates. As expected, these differences in metabolite profiles could be explained by the increased metabolism of plant-derived complex sugar molecules by the vegan group's gut microbiota, and the increased amount of animal-related amino acids and lipids consumed by the omnivores.

In short, diet changed the study subjects' production of microbial metabolites without significantly changing the composition of the microorganisms that produced these metabolites. The investigators speculated that if diet is the reason for the significant differences in gut microbiota previously observed in distinct human populations in different parts of the world, then such diet-related differences may take several generations to evolve or may require very early life exposures to have a lasting effect on the gut microbiota.

We now know that there are multiple mechanisms by which the gut microbiota can be influenced early in life, including the mother's diet in pregnancy and during nursing, exposure to environmental microbes, and stress-induced brain-gut signals that affect both the mother and the infant's gut microbiomes. The geographic differences in microbiota composition may also be due in part to the major differences in the environmental conditions of individuals living in harmony with their environment in isolated parts of the world, compared to those of American city dwellers living in metropolitan areas, removed from direct exposure to natural environments and getting their food from the supermarket or restaurants.

Despite the adaptability of our microbiota, it's also true that the microbiota of rural agrarians and hunter-gatherers have capabilities that we have simply lost. Even if we decided to start eating the same diet as a hunter-gatherer or traditional rural agrarian, we'd never be able to ferment plant food as well or produce as many useful metabolites in our gut as they do. This so-called permissive microbiota produces an abundant supply of short-chain fatty acids—energy-rich beneficial molecules that may protect against colon cancer and inflammatory bowel disease and are likely to play a role in gut-to-brain communication.

People living in industrialized societies, in contrast, have a "restrictive" gut microbiota composition that is not as efficient in fermenting complex plant-based carbohydrates to short-chain fatty acids, even if you consume a lot of fruits, vegetables, and other plant-derived foods. How would such a restrictive composition develop?

Wu thinks that this may be due to the absence of certain microbial species, such as the bacterium *Ruminococcus bromii*, whose activities are essential for initiating the degradation of these hard-to-break-down substrates. Within the ecosystem of the gut microbiome, many of the same metabolites can be produced by different members of the microbial community and are consumed or transformed by others. On the other hand, other species of gut microbes have more specialized skills, and appear to play a key role in degrading starch particles that escape digestion in the small intestine. This so-called resistant starch is contained in a wide variety of plant-based foods, including bananas, potatoes, seeds, legumes, and unprocessed whole grains. In most individuals, resistant starch is completely fermented to short-chain fatty acids in the colon, but some people's gut microbiota lack that ability.

It turns out that *Ruminococcus bromii* will typically initiate the breakdown of resistant starch, making the partially digested substrate available to other bacteria, which then break down the individual sugars further using different enzymes. Microorganisms like *Ruminococcus bromii* are known in ecological parlance as a "keystone species," as they carry out activities that are essential for the ecosystem as a whole to function optimally. Wolves, for example, are keystone species in Yellowstone National Park, where they control the population of elk, which keeps the elk from overgrazing and thereby keeps the ecosystem in balance. A disappearance of wolves has widespread consequences on a large number of downstream species and ultimately will affect the function of the entire ecosystem. In the gut microbiome, all of the other microbes are compromised in their ability to do their job (such as metabolizing complex carbohydrates) if a keystone species like *Ruminococcus bromii* is reduced or absent. In contrast, if any of the downstream species should be absent, their work can readily be taken over by other downstream actors.

All this means that when you are born into Western civilization, you acquire a Western microbiome as well. Even if you go vegan today, your gut microbiota will remain that of a typical omnivore, and even if you eat a paleo diet for the rest of your life, your gut microbiota won't turn into that of a hunter-gatherer. However, the pattern of microbial metabolites you produce depends on which diet you consume.

That said, even if you and a neighbor eat a very similar diet, you will have different species of microbes in your gut than she does. We only share a small amount of the microbial species and strains with our fellow humans, even though we look pretty similar in terms of the genes these microbes express and the metabolites that they produce. As Rob Knight, at the University of California, San Diego, whose analytical genius has made modern gut microbiome research possible, puts it, the gut microbiome is like a large-scale ecosystem in which different groupings of microbial species can carry out the same functions. While two grasslands might look similar in a picture, especially when compared to two forests, the two grasslands may well differ in the hundreds of plant and animal species that live in them and that create these similar-appearing environments.

If you are a music lover, you may visualize the relationship between the composition of your gut microbiota and their functions in a different way. You probably have your favorite orchestra, like the Los Angeles or Berlin philharmonic, which you have listened to many times. Most of the musicians in these orchestras have been the same every time you have listened to one of their concerts, yet the music they play, be it a symphony by Beethoven, Mahler, or Mozart, is completely different depending on the notes the musicians are given. So when it comes to your health, the identity of the microbial species matters less than the job that they do, just as the identity of the individual musicians is less important to your enjoyment than the piece of music they play.

How Diet Changes the Gut-Brain Conversation

As Wu's study illustrates, our gut microbiota can adapt to dramatic changes in our food sources by changing the food they live on, and the metabolites they produce. This is one element of the enormous evolutionary wisdom contained in the gut. We've discussed how this wisdom has been programmed into our gut-microbiome-brain axis, and how it has provided us with not only a perfectly functioning digestive system, but also a growing library of gut feelings that help us predict the future, and instincts that help tune our awareness to the dangers in our world. Importantly, while our gut microbiome along with its connection with the brain is programmed early in life, it also remains flexible and adaptable throughout life.

Throughout this book I've described our brain-gut-microbiome axis as analogous to a supercomputer—one that can perfectly adjust to the ongoing changes in our internal and external world, and that has intricate connections to our immune system, our metabolism, our nervous system, and every other system in our body. The adaptability of the gut-brain-microbiome axis is clearly demonstrated by the fact that humans were able (until recently) to transition successfully from the prehistoric lifestyle, which was closely connected with the natural environment, to a lifestyle in which we live in megacities and eat food items that often come from distant regions across the world. Our gut microbiome can even learn to metabolize substances it has never encountered before, including many of the modern drugs, pesticides, and chemicals that we ingest.

Because of this versatility, there's good reason to assume that your gut metabolites will differ depending on what type of diet you eat. That's because the breakdown of complex plant-derived carbohydrates, such as resistant starch, generates a fundamentally different set of metabolites than the breakdown of amino acids and fats—major components of meat and milk, eggs, and cheese. For example, in contrast to the rather limited range of carbohydrate metabolites—which consist primarily of just a few short-chain fatty acids—your body digests proteins into twenty different building-block molecules, called amino acids, and microbes in the colon ferment these amino acids into a much wider range of metabolites, which can interact with the nervous system.

Most undigested plant-derived carbohydrates are metabolized by microbes in the colon into short-chain fatty acids such as butyrate—so named because it has a buttery odor—and acetate, as well as gases such as carbon dioxide, methane, and hydrogen sulfide (which gives stool a bad odor). Butyrate is an excellent example of the many health-promoting effects of plant-based diets on the health of the gut-brain axis. It not only plays a crucial role in providing food for the cells lining the colon, preventing it from becoming leaky, but also has many health-promoting effects on the enteric nervous system. And this short-chain fatty acid represents a key player in the communication between the gut and the brain in the regulation of food intake, in particular in creating a feeling of satiety which causes us to stop eating beyond our body's needs. Butyrate interacts with specialized molecules located on the hormone-containing cells in our gut, so-called short-chain fatty acid receptors, making these cells release their content into the circulation and onto adjacent sensory nerve endings of the vagus nerve. These gut-brain signals are crucial in telling our brain when it is time to stop eating.

Illustrating the tremendous potential that changes in diet can have on your brain, it has been estimated that the human gut microbiome has the potential to produce some 500,000 distinct metabolites, known collectively as the metabolome, and many of these metabolites are neuroactive, which means they can influence your nervous system. Some individual microorganisms produce up to fifty different metabolites, including hormones, neurotransmitters, and other molecules that communicate directly with the nervous system. There can also be up to 40,000 variations of any given metabolite, depending on how it's combined with other metabolites. These metabolites are produced by some 7 million genes, far more than the 20,000 in the human genome.

Since we eat such a diversity of foods, particularly plant foods, and our guts contain such vast numbers of diverse microbial cells, it has been estimated that 40 percent of the metabolites circulating in our bodies are produced not by our own cells and tissues, but instead by our gut microbes. Indeed, it's becoming clear that your gut microbiome plays a key role in a remarkably complex signaling system that can influence every cell in your body, including those in the brain. Although it will take years of research to untangle all the complex effects that these microbial metabolites have on us—either by themselves or more likely in combination with others—there is no question in my mind that these effects are profound and will revolutionize the way we understand the role of diet in the development and in the treatment of disorders of the brain and the brain-gut axis. In other words, the orchestra of microbes in your gut is fully staffed with seasoned musicians, and ready to perform from the first years of life. The diet you choose determines not only the tunes it plays, but also the quality of these tunes. And you, ultimately, are the conductor of the symphony.

9

THE ONSLAUGHT OF THE NORTH AMERICAN DIET: WHAT EVOLUTION DID NOT FORESEE

It was one of those days. You overslept, rushed out of the house without breakfast, got stuck in rush hour traffic, and arrived at work thirty minutes late, missing the beginning of an important meeting. In order to make up for your late arrival, you stayed at your desk for an extra hour and weren't able to pick up your daughter from soccer practice, earning you the resentment of both your wife and daughter. When your frantic day finally came to a close, you left the office at six, stopping at a gas station on the way home to fill up your near-empty tank. While you were there you grabbed a bag of chips and a candy bar and devoured them in the car. By the time you pulled into your driveway, your mood had lifted a little.

Many of us can relate to a scenario like this—on a day when

we're feeling particularly stressed or anxious, we reach for foods—donuts, bagels, muffins, candy—that make us feel a little better. Our emotional states are closely related to our fat and sugar intake, and many of us aren't paying enough attention to what we're eating. In fact, more than 35 percent of calories in the American diet comes from fat, most of it from animal sources. Even though the standard diet in several northern European and even Mediterranean countries (like Greece) have a similar total fat intake, the North American diet stands out in terms of animal fat consumption, with a significantly higher percentage of animal fat compared to the Mediterranean diet. It's well known that this excessive animal fat intake, together with excessive sugar intake, is a contributing factor to the American obesity epidemic. But it's perhaps less well known that a diet high in animal fat can also contribute to overconsumption of food and even food addiction—and our gut microbes may play an important role in this connection. On the other hand, recent epidemiological evidence suggest that diets low in animal fat, such as the Mediterranean diet, don't just have positive consequences for your waistline, metabolism, and cardiovascular health. Such diets are also associated with a lower risk for certain cancers and serious brain diseases such as depression, Alzheimer's, and Parkinson's disease.

Studies in animals and humans have demonstrated that a key link between the overconsumption of animal fats and the onset of disease—including diseases of the brain—is a chronic state of low-grade inflammation. Inflammation that starts in the gut can spread throughout the body, reaching crucial brain regions (including those that control our appetite). Our gut microbes play a key role in this process. In this way, our modern North American diet—high in animal fat, low in plants, and enriched with chemicals and preservatives—is reprogramming our gut-brain-microbiome axis, and not for the better.

Taken together with the disturbing changes in our agricultural and food processing methods, this shift in our diet has led to what can only be called a watershed moment in human physiology—an extremely dangerous one.

Our Brave New Diet

We've discussed how, throughout our evolution, humans have been able to switch easily between diets high in animal protein and those rich in plants, depending on which foods were available. For that we can thank our gut microbes, their vast number of genes, and their sophisticated ability to detect substances in our food and transform them into beneficial metabolites, thereby adjusting our own metabolism and food intake to accommodate our changing diet. But as we have seen in the eating habits of the Yanomami or the Hazda, our ancestors evolved in an environment of not only a limited and hard-to-obtain food supply, but also the near absence of foods high in fat and refined sugars. In other words, evolution never anticipated the standard American diet of today. And our gut-microbiome brain axis is ill prepared to come with the consequences of that diet.

If you think of your digestive system as a turbine engine that can burn any type of combustible material to generate energy, it automatically follows that you should be able to digest and metabolize whatever you want. In fact, this "engine" metaphor is of critical importance to the food industry. Millions of consumers are willing to buy anything labeled as "food," as long as it can be packaged into a shape, taste, and smell that appeals. But if we think of our brain-gut-microbiome axis as an information-processing supercomputer that constantly tries to adjust our behavior and our bodies to ongoing changes in our internal and external world, then we can understand what's happening today.

In recent decades, changes fueled by the profit-driven activities of corporations involved in the production, processing, and marketing of inexpensive, highly addictive foods have completely altered our diet. This in turn has directly affected the interactions between our brains, our guts, and the microbiome. Strangely, this has not only happened to our own bodies but has also occurred in our livestock (and in our pets) as well.

We know that our gut microbiome has no problem rapidly switching between animal- or plant-based diets. In fact, the omnivore diet (which was practiced by our prehistoric ancestors for hundreds of thousands of years) may actually be our default diet, with the vegetarian diet being a fallback solution for times when the availability of animal products was limited. But today's animal products are fundamentally different from what our ancestors ate, and what their few remaining direct descendants, living in isolated prehistoric societies, continue to eat. The meat that these primal people eat is drawn from many different animal species—including wild animals and birds, fish, and insects—and it's lean, with dramatically lower fat content than today's commercial meat products. These animals roam free and unrestrained in natural environments, feeding on a vast variety of plants and other creatures. They have an intact, highly diverse gut microbiome, making them healthy and resistant to diseases.

It's clear that the increased availability of animal protein has had significant benefits. It has played a major role in enabling our brains to grow larger over the course of human evolution, and it has helped increase our average height over the past century.

But in contrast to our ancestors' protein supply, our livestock often live out their lives in small pens, eating feed (like corn) that their digestive systems are not built to handle, and which is designed to fatten them as efficiently as possible. They ingest antibiotics and other chemicals, which reduce the diversity of their gut microbes and make them more vulnerable to serious gut infections. For all these reasons, the meat, eggs, and milk that come from these animals—and derivatives of these products (often no longer recognizable as food) in today's processed food—are dramatically different from only fifty years ago, and they have fundamentally altered our diet.

Unfortunately, evolution hasn't had enough time to program our defenses against these changes, and as a result, our brave new food supply has caught our bodies unprepared. It is only recently that people have become aware of these dangers and begun to take action.

How a Diet High in Animal Fat Can Harm Your Brain

Why does our modern diet, supplied in large part by today's food industry, damage our bodies and brains? There are several factors that have been implicated as the major culprit in the dysregulation of gut microbiome brain affecting our health, including the excessive consumption of sugar and the insufficient intake of dietary fiber. However, in the following, I will focus on one of the strongest body of evidence coming both from studies in animals and human populations supporting the detrimental role of high consumption of fat from animal sources as part of the North American diet.

For years, scientists have linked chronic disease to overweight and obesity. As the theory went, fat cells in our body, particularly fat stores in our belly (so called visceral fat), were the primary source of inflammatory molecules, called cyto-kines or adipokines, that circulate in the blood, reaching the heart, the liver, and the brain. These inflammatory molecules were thought to be the chief cause of low-grade inflammation, also known as "metabolic endotoxemia," which in turn raised the risk of cardiovascular disease and cancer. Brain diseases such as depression, Alzheimer's, and Parkinson's were rarely brought into context with these peripheral metabolic processes.

According to this theory, as long as your weight was in the normal range and your waistline hadn't increased, you could continue indulging in your bacon for breakfast, your hamburg-ers and hot dogs and fat-laden tortilla chips, without any ill effects.

But it is now clear that even a single high-fat meal can switch your gut's immune system into the low-grade inflammation mode and that regular consumption of a diet high in animal fat can trigger persistent low-grade inflammation long before a person becomes obese. A single time of switching on your gut's immune system, such as when you gobble down a deli-cious piece of cheesecake or a chocolate sundae after dinner, is unlikely to cause any ill effects on your brain. However, when you regularly consume foods packed with animal fats, it is a more serious story.

Today, there's far more animal fat hidden in all the things we love to eat, and while we are craving and enjoying the con-sumption of these tasty meals, they secretly manipulate our gut microbiota, their metabolites, and our eating behavior. In order to understand how this manipulation occurs, we have to briefly recall how the gut-brain axis normally regulates our food intake.

The language that signals your brain to stop eating when you've eaten enough and feel hungry again when your stom-ach is empty includes hormones that can stimulate or turn off your appetite, the latter being called satiety hormones. These gut hormones target a brain region called the hypothalamus, which is the master regulator of our eating behavior. When the system is working properly, the hypothalamus can precisely compute how many calories your body needs on any given day, based on your level of physical activity, the temperature, and other factors that influence your metabolism. The hypothalamus is one of the most widely connected regions in the brain, reflecting its ability to collect vast amounts of vital information and to influence other regions of the brain. A large portion of this information comes from the gut, sent in the form of various gut hormones and vagal nerve signals.

When you're hungry, enteroendocrine cells interspersed within the cells lining your stomach release a hormone, called ghrelin, also known as the hunger hormone, which either travels through the bloodstream to the brain or stimulates the tips of the vagus nerve in the gut to signal the brain directly. On the other hand, when you've had enough to eat, a different group of appetite-suppressing hormones (including cholecystokinin and glucagon-like peptide) are released from enteroendocrine cells in your small intestine, and these hormones turn the system off and suppress appetite.

For most of mankind's existence, this system has worked remarkably well, keeping our weights surprisingly stable over the long term, despite dramatic fluctuations in food intake and physical activity. It has kept us alive through prolonged droughts and famines, and through the transition from prehistoric diets through the meals common in the antiquities all the way to modern diets of today. For many in the United States, however, it no longer does, and these changes in appetite regulation that have occurred in the last fifty years play a major role in our current obesity epidemic

What exactly happened to cause your appetite-control system to stop working properly?

Over the past few years, investigators have been looking hard for answers. We know now from animal experiments that a regular high-fat diet can numb the satiety response both at the gut and the brain level, reducing your ability to tell when you've eaten enough. There is solid evidence that it does this in both locations by causing low-grade inflammation. In the gut, that inflammation reduces sensitivity to satiety signals by sensors on the vagus nerve, which normally tell your hypothalamus that you're full. In your hypothalamus, it reduces sensitivity to satiety signals arriving from the gut.

But how does diet cause inflammation in the first place? As new science is now revealing, your gut microbiota play a pivotal role.

How Your Gut Microbes Help Regulate Appetite

When you ingest a high-fat meal, blood levels of inflammatory molecules increase throughout your body. These include cytokines and a substance called lipopolysaccharide (LPS), which is part of the cell wall of certain gut microbiota known as gram-negative bacteria. Gram-negative bacteria include many pathogens, such as *E. coli* and salmonella, but also many of the dominant groups of microbiota living in our gut, including the phyla of Firmicutes and Proteobacteria, whose populations rise when we eat a diet heavy in animal fat. When a gut microbe approaches the cells that line the inner gut, these cells recognize LPS on the microbe's surface and use a receptor to bind it. LPS stimulates these cells to produce other inflammatory molecules (cytokines), makes the gut leakier, and activates the immune cells in the gut.

Under normal conditions, as discussed in Chapter 6, several barriers prevent LPS and other microbial inflammatory signals from initiating this sequence of events. As LPS levels increase (as they do in response to a high-animal-fat diet), the molecule starts to breach these barriers and activate the gut's immune system to produce cytokines and reach distant sites within our bodies, including our brain. Once these molecules reach the brain, they get access to its immune system, the glial cells, which start producing inflammatory molecules themselves, targeting nearby nerve cells in the brain. In the hypothalamus, such inflammatory changes make this appetite-regulating center less responsive to the satiety signals from the gut and the body.

Several other lines of evidence further support the notion that gut microbes play a central role when a high-fat diet causes systemic inflammation. A few years ago, microbiome expert Andrew Gewirtz, at Georgia State University, genetically removed a different class of toll-like receptors involved in the innate immune response. Animals lacking the receptors become obese and develop all the features of metabolic syndrome, a constellation of resistance to the hormone insulin, increased blood sugar levels, and increased triglycerides. The weight gain of the animals was related to their voracious appetite, suggesting a defect in their satiety mechanisms.

Then the researchers found something particularly intriguing. These obese, genetically modified mice had a different mix of gut microbes than normal mice, and when Gewirtz's team transplanted their stool into lean germ-free mice, the lean animals developed the same metabolic features as the donor mice. Most important, they also developed the same uninhibited food intake and became obese. It's plausible that the changes in the animals' gut microbiota and their altered interactions with their gut-based innate immune system led to a state of metabolic toxemia, the low-grade systemic inflammation discussed earlier. Once these inflammatory signals reach the hypothalamus, the appetite-controlling mechanism is thrown off balance.

A high-fat diet is not only able to change the inner workings of the hypothalamus to change your appetite, but also is likely to compromise appetite regulation by altering some of the key appetite-related sensors in the gut wall itself. Neuroscientist Helen Raybould's group at the University of California, Davis, asked the question if changes in a high-fat diet can change the relative sensitivity of vagal sensory nerve endings in the gut to appetite-stimulating and appetite-suppressing gut signals, and if these changes are associated with a compromised inhibition of food intake. They had previously shown that the satiety hormone cholecystokinin, released by cells in the gut in the presence of fat, was able to switch these nerve endings from a "hunger mode" to a "satiety mode." The investigators showed that feeding rats a high-fat diet for eight weeks made some of them overeat and gain weight. This excessive eating was associated with an increase in receptors on vagal sensors in the gut for food-stimulating signals and the development of resistance to the hormone leptin, which reduces appetite.

The Lure of Comfort Foods

If low-grade inflammation can compromise our appetite mechanisms and negatively affect our brain and our gut, why is it that we crave unhealthy, fat-containing foods when we are under stress? Why don't we nibble on carrots and apples when we're stuck in traffic or stressed out over a looming deadline?

A small number of studies performed in animals and in healthy human subjects have identified possible mechanisms for this stress-reducing effect of fatty and sugary foods. For example, several laboratories had shown that chronically stressed rats showed a down-regulation of their stress system when they were allowed to eat high-fat or sugary drinks, compared to those given no such "comfort foods." Similarly, when adult rats who had experienced early life adversity (the stressful maternal separation paradigm after they were born) were allowed to eat a highly palatable, high-fat diet, this eating pattern actually reversed the up-regulation of their stress response system and reduced their anxiety- and depression-like behaviors. Inspired by the findings of these mouse studies, several investigators explored whether human subjects experience similar positive effects from eating comfort food when they're stressed or in a negative emotional state.

Janet Tomiyama and her team in the Department of Psychology at UCLA investigated whether the stress responsiveness of healthy subjects to an acute laboratory stressor was related to a history of higher consumption of comfort foods after stressful events, and also whether this was reflected in a greater degree of obesity. They based their hypothesis on the fact that animals accumulate fat in the belly area through repeated consumption of highly palatable foods, which in turn leads to inhibition of the stress response system in chronically stressed animals. To test their theory, they exposed fifty-nine healthy women to a stressful laboratory task. They measured levels of the stress hormone cortisol in the subjects' blood and charted their subjective experience of stress while performing the task. Consistent with the researchers' hypothesis and the animal literature, the women who had the lowest stress ratings and the lowest cortisol response were the most likely to report a history of stress-related eating of comfort food and also had the greatest degree of obesity. Even though other explanations of these findings are possible, they suggest that women who regularly eat comfort foods when stressed dampen their physiological response to stress. Unfortunately, this food-induced stress reduction comes at the cost of weight gain and all the other detrimental changes in our bodies and brains.

Lukas Van Oudenhove, a psychiatrist at the University of Leuven in Belgium, studied subjective reports and brain responses using fMRI (functional magnetic resonance imaging) in healthy volunteers to evaluate the effect of fat ingestion on a variety of subjective parameters, including personal ratings of mood, and responses in specific emotional brain regions. A feeling of sadness or neutrality was induced by having subjects listen for thirty minutes to sad or neutral classical music while at the same time being shown images of faces expressing sad or neutral emotions. Fat was then infused directly into the stomach of the experimental subjects via a small plastic feeding tube, while water was infused in other subjects as a control condition. The ratings of mood and the activation of the emotional brain regions during the negative stimulus clearly demonstrated both an increase of feelings of sadness and an increase in brain reactions. When the subjects received the infusion of fatty acids into their stomach, both the subjective feelings of sadness and the associated emotional brain responses were reduced—supporting the idea that high fat intake can have an emotionally comforting effect. We have already learned how the gut, its enteroendocrine cells, and the vagus nerve respond to the presence of fat in the small intestine. Based on these interactions, we can speculate that the fatty acids improved the subjects' mood by stimulating the release of signaling molecules from the gut, which reached emotional brain regions via the circulation or via increased signaling of the vagus nerve.

Unfortunately, the ill effects of unhealthy eating habits on our brain and behavior are not limited to appetite control and our responses to stress. Recent scientific evidence has linked such habits to even more serious consequences of altered brain function.

Food Addiction: The Effect of a High-Fat, High-Sugar Diet on Food Cravings

While the term "addictive behavior" is generally used in connection to drugs and alcohol as well as compulsive sexual behaviors, the term has recently been applied to the eating of food in general, and also to the consumption of specific foods such as sugar. We now know that in some vulnerable individuals, food may evoke psychopharmacological and behavioral responses similar to those produced by repeated use of other stimulants.

How much food you eat is controlled by three closely interacting systems in your brain: in addition to the appetite control system regulated by the hypothalamus, there are two other brain systems that play a prominent role: the dopamine reward system, and the executive control system, located in your brain's prefrontal cortex, which can voluntarily override all other control systems if needed. In the world of hunter-gatherers, characterized by limited food supplies and high energy needs, the urge to eat was driven by the constant existential need of their bodies for food (experienced subjectively as a gut feeling of hunger). This basic caloric needs assessment system was assisted by the reward system, providing the drive and motivation to search for food. Dopamine-containing nerves, which make up large portions of the brain's reward network, promise a major reward if we pursue a certain action. They play a major role in modulating the motivation and sustainability of behaviors necessary to obtain the reward, in this case the drive and motivation to forage for food.

Not surprisingly, there are very close connections between the brain's reward system and the networks involved in appetite regulation. For example, a number of gut hormones and signaling molecules influence activity in the dopaminergic reward pathway: several appetite-boosting signals increase the activity of dopamine-containing cells, while certain appetite-suppressing signals decrease dopamine release. In addition, nerve cells in key regions of the reward system, such as the nucleus accumbens, express receptors for various gut hormones involved in appetite regulation: appetite-suppressing hormones, such as leptin, peptide YY, and glucagon-like peptide, decrease the sensitivity of the reward system, while appetite-stimulating hormones such as insulin and ghrelin increase it.

Millions of years of evolution have optimized this elaborate interaction between reward and appetite for a world of limited and difficult-to-obtain food supplies, a situation that has existed for the great majority of human existence on this planet. However, this hardwiring of our brain systems related to food intake loses much of its adaptive value in the world most of us inhabit today. In our modern industrialized society, with its easy access to highly palatable food and dramatically reduced levels of physical activity, the drive of the reward system can easily overwhelm the control system computing our daily caloric needs, and often has to be controlled voluntarily to avoid overeating and weight gain. Now imagine a scenario in which one of these control systems has been switched off and there is a limited capacity of voluntary control mechanisms to make up for it. This is exactly the situation I described earlier when explaining how chronic high fat intake can compromise the hypothalamus's ability to respond to satiety signals from the gut. Not everybody has the discipline to say "no" to a side dish of french fries, or when shown the dessert menu in a restaurant!

One of the behaviors that can result from this remodeling of our appetite control mechanisms is food addiction. This term was coined by Nora Volkow, director of the National Institute on Drug Abuse, based on the astonishing neurobiological similarities between the brain mechanisms that underlie substance abuse and chronic overeating. Based on questionnaire data, it's estimated that at least 20 percent of obese individuals suffer from food addiction. Certain foods, especially high-calorie foods rich in fat and sugar, have been shown to trigger addictive eating behavior in both animals and humans. Our own group's work at UCLA has identified structural and functional changes in key regions of the brain's reward system among overweight and obese (but otherwise healthy) subjects. These mechanisms not only promote overeating but also produce learned associations, also known as conditioned responses, between the stimulus of the food and the reward signals in the brain. The prime importance of these conditioned responses is the reason our living rooms are flooded with TV commercials showing images of food that is both highly palatable and high in fat. In most people these images will stimulate the brain's reward system, which has been programmed throughout evolution to seek out foods with high caloric density, in particular fat and refined sugars. This reaction on its own is a desirable outcome for advertisers, since it instills a positive conditioned response to their products. In individuals who suffer from food addiction, however (and in whom the normal appetite control system has been compromised by a low-grade inflammatory state), viewing these images will actually create a craving to go to the kitchen, or to pick up the phone and order such foods for home delivery.

In times when food was scarce and an animal had to maximally take advantage of any situation that provided access to food, this ability of palatable foods to stimulate overconsumption— and to encode strong memories that increase our cravings for them—had major evolutionary advantages. Among other things, it helped ensure that we splurged on these calorie-rich sources when we found them, and that we remembered where to find them in the future. In environments where such foods are plentiful and ubiquitous, however—as it is in many parts of the world today—this property has become a dangerous liability. In modern society, palatable foods, like drugs of abuse, represent a powerful environmental trigger, which can facilitate or exacerbate uncontrolled eating behavior in vulnerable individuals.

As explained earlier, there is good evidence that the dominance of hedonic food seeking may be caused by the inactivation of the hypothalamic control system by the metabolic toxemia. But there's also recent evidence suggesting that such unrestricted activity of the reward system in food-addicted individuals may further compromise gut function. In a recent study of individuals suffering from alcohol dependence, it was shown that cravings for alcohol during periods of abstinence were positively correlated with the individuals' intestinal permeability (how leaky their guts were) and with changes in their gut microbiota. Given the strong engagement of the brain's stress response during craving and the well-known effects of stress on gut permeability, it's conceivable that the permeability effects in this study were related to a craving-related (and stress-related) increase in the gut's leakiness and the observed changes in gut microbial composition and metabolic function.

The idea that our gut microbes may influence our reward system and play a role in food addiction has led to many speculations about the relationship between ourselves and our gut microbiome, even questioning the idea of free will. In a provocative review article, Joe Alcock, a professor at the University of Mexico, recently suggested that gut microbes may be under strong selective pressure to manipulate human eating behavior in ways that increase their own fitness, sometimes at the expense of our health. This hypothesis is not as far-fetched as it may seem at first glance; we only need to remember the sophisticated ways that some microbial organisms, such as the *Toxoplasma gondii* parasite, can manipulate the behavior of animals. Alcock and his coauthors proposed that gut microbes might do this through two potential interacting strategies. On the one hand, by hijacking our dopamine-driven reward system, they may be able to generate cravings for particular foods that they are specialized to consume and that give them an advantage over competitive microbial species. A good example would be the competitions between microbial groups of the Bacteroidetes and Firmicutes taxa and between Bacterioides and Prevotella. Second, they may create negative mood states—causing us to feel depressed, for example—that don't go away until we eat certain food components that benefit these gut microbes.

The drive to eat so-called comfort food and the concept of food addiction are both excellent examples of behaviors that could potentially be manipulated by certain types of gut microbiota to provide them with their preferred foods. While these concepts currently belong to the realm of speculative science, that is, speculations based on incomplete scientific evidence, they are intriguing hypotheses that will need to be tested scientifically in the future.

If you are not already worried enough about your diet—there's more. Fat is far from the only threat to your brain-gut-microbiome axis lurking in the North American diet. And as we will learn, the gut microbes play an important role in this threat.

How Industrial Agriculture Affects Your Gut and Brain

Growing up in the Bavarian Alps, hardly a summer weekend went by when my dad and I weren't hiking in the local mountains. Watching the cows grazing on grassy alpine meadows sprinkled with wildflowers was a familiar experience. Yet, at the time, I didn't pay much attention to it, and I had no clue that I would once return to these childhood images with important scientific questions. The farmers would sell unpasteurized milk in small mountain restaurants directly from these happy and healthy-looking animals. All the dairy products that we ate in our family came from these animals roaming free in the mountains, and there was a general awareness that every product that came from them was natural, healthy, and delicious.

When I spoke at a gastroenterology conference in Garmisch, an idyllic resort town at the bottom of Bavaria's highest mountain, the Zugspitze, I had another chance to look at this harmonious relationship between the farm animals and their environment, this time with very different eyes. While taking a train to reach the top of the mountain for my talk, I looked at these animals grazing on pristine meadows surrounded by patches of trees in glowing fall colors. I couldn't help contrasting these images of natural harmony with the desolate existence of cows on a modern cattle feedlot, which I had seen in Northern California. Such images give the lie to advertisements from industrial dairies about milk from "happy cows." In his book *The Missing Microbes*, Martin Blaser provides a more accurate picture of the modern cattle feedlot:

Cows lined up in small metal pens, row after row of them, with their heads braced into corn-filled troughs. A dense, pungent odor of cow manure wafts from miles away. Cows are released into vast feedlots where they mill around on bare ground, eating all the time, surrounded by their poop.

Indeed, today's farm animals are kept completely separate from their natural environments and food supplies (grass) for most of their lives. Fattening of the animals with corn, a food source unsuitable for the cows' digestive system, leads to diseases of their digestive system, resulting in a chronic, low-grade inflammatory state and often superimposed acute gastrointestinal infections that require continual administration of antibiotics.

From what we know about the effect of an unhealthy diet and of chronic stress on the gut microbes, the gut-based immune system, and the leakiness of the gut, we can't escape the suspicions that the products that come from such chronically diseased animals are not good for our gut microbiota and not beneficial for our health. So the next time you buy milk, eggs, steak, or pork chops in the supermarket, be aware that they probably came from animals whose brain-gut-microbiome axis has been severely modified by the deplorable conditions in which they're raised, the chronic stress that is associated with these living conditions, the unnatural diet they've been fed (not suitable for their digestive system), and the medications they've received—all of which pose unknown risks for the optimal function of our gut-microbiota-brain interactions and for our own health.

Sadly, the situation is not much better in regard to the vegetables, fruits, and other plant-based foods. A common theme shared by animal- and plant-based food production is the massive interference of the corporate agribusiness with the ecology of farm animals, plants, and microbial organisms. Industrial farming of corn, soybeans, and wheat is heavily dependent on fertilizers and pesticides, used to artificially maintain the growth and dominance of these plants over competitive plant species such as weeds and to defend them against pests and harmful insects. The use of systemic insecticides, which are ultimately incorporated and expressed in the entire plant and its products, has greatly increased in the last decade.

One of the key reasons why ever-increasing amounts of chemicals are needed to maintain the "health" and dominance of these plants is the fact that these monocultures of often genetically modified single-crop fields, stretching across the landscape for miles, have completely lost their natural diversity in terms of both the genetic variety of the crops themselves and the variety of other species that coexist with them. It's highly likely that equally drastic changes are occurring in the diversity of microorganisms living in the soil, in the gut microbiomes of the declining bee and butterfly populations, and in the microbes living in our own gastrointestinal tract. Along the same lines, the collateral damage on our gut microbiome of the increasing deployment of weed killers (such as the notorious glyphosate, or "Roundup")—necessary to overcome the weeds' resistance to such chemicals—remains largely unknown, at least to the consumer.

One important question is whether this dual chemical insult on the natural ecosystems of our environment (where our food comes from) and on the internal gut microbial ecosystems of our farm animals and ourselves (which play a major role in maintaining the health of our brains) is contributing to the dramatic increases in certain brain diseases over the past fifty years. While the scientific evidence to answer this question is already available for obesity, we can only speculate at the moment if this also applies to autism spectrum disorders and neurodegenerative disorders such as Alzheimer's and Parkinson's disease. If this question is left to the corporate world, which benefits daily from these unsustainable practices of food production, we'll never get an answer. Instead we will continue to be caught in a spiral of ever-increasing doses of antibiotics to keep farm animals functioning, and chemicals needed to fight today's superweeds, superbugs, and supergerms.

Gut Microbes and the Dangers of the Modern American Diet

Over the past fifty years, Americans have not only consumed steadily increasing amounts of food additives but salt, sugar, and fat. Many of them were approved for human use without being tested for their long-term safety. And even when they were, they were tested before we had learned how important the gut microbiome was to our health, and what intermediary effect they can play between these additives and our brain health. Safety tests used by the U.S. Food and Drug Administration (FDA) have largely relied on short-term animal models that were designed to detect whether the additive had a fast-acting toxic effect, whether it heightened the risk of cancer, or both. None of these short-term tests are able to inform us about the possible detrimental effects of such additives on long-term brain health

Today we know that several of the most common types of additives contribute to the low-grade inflammatory state in our bodies that, along with our high fat and sugar intake, endangers our bodies and our brains. Let's look at them one by one.

Artificial Sweeteners

One of the best examples of the extreme changes that have occurred in our diet due to food additives is the way the food industry has responded to our insatiable appetite for sugars. On the one side, vast amounts of sugar have been added to a wide range of foods in the form of high-fructose corn syrup, even to food items (like breads and crackers) that we don't seek out to satisfy our sweet tooth. On the other hand, artificial sweeteners have been added to just about anything we seek out to reconcile our cravings for sweet taste with our concern about calories. Introduced more than a century ago, artificial sweeteners were developed to let us enjoy sweet foods without the weight gain and hazardous spikes in blood sugar caused by high sugar intake. If artificial sweeteners came with mottos, it would be "you can have your cake and eat it too." The FDA has approved six such substances for use in the United States. Today these chemicals are added in massive amounts to commonly consumed foods such as diet sodas, cereals, and sugar-free desserts. And they remain popular, even among the scientifically savvy. At the noon medical conferences in my department at UCLA, Diet Coke and Diet Pepsi remain the most popular beverage choices with lunch (not to mention the pastrami sandwiches, full of processed meat) and the greasy potato chips.

Despite their ubiquity, evidence for their promised health benefits is mixed at best, and evidence for dangers of artificial sweeteners has emerged, including weight gain and increased risk of metabolic diseases such as type 2 diabetes. For example, Jotham Suez's group at the Weizmann Institute of Science in Jerusalem showed recently that three commercially available sweeteners—saccharin, sucralose, and aspartame—can induce glucose intolerance and signs of metabolic syndrome in mice. These findings are intriguing enough by themselves, but what is even more intriguing is their discovery that the gut microbiota played a major role in this effect. Suez's team proved this conclusion by transplanting stool from mice that consumed artificial sweeteners into germ-free mice that had never eaten sweeteners, causing the formerly germ-free mice to develop glucose intolerance and signs of metabolic syndrome. By analyzing the animals' microbiota, they noticed that consuming artificial sweetener led Bacteroides bacteria to flourish in the animals' gut, just as a high-fat diet does. This means that far from helping you lose weight, a diet soda with that fatty cheesy enchilada could exacerbate the harm all the fat in that cheese is doing to your metabolism.

The researchers also showed that sweeteners changed metabolic pathways in gut microbes so they produce more short-chain fatty acids, which can be absorbed by the colon, providing additional calories. This means that when you consume artificial sweeteners, your body enlists your gut microbiota to harvest more calories in the colon from the microbial metabolic products to compensate for the missing sugar available in the small intestine. It suggests that trying to cut calories with artificial sweeteners won't work because your gut, with the help of its microbes, will just extract proportionally more calories from the food you eat.

The results held for human subjects, too. When Suez's group tested several hundred human subjects, they found that individuals who consumed artificial sweeteners were heavier, had higher fasting blood sugar levels, and had altered gut microbiota as well. And their gut microbiota were clearly responsible. When the investigators transplanted stool from healthy, saccharin-consuming subjects into germ-free mice, eating sugar began causing the animals' blood sugar to spike to abnormal levels.

These studies provide strong evidence that artificial sweeteners not only fail to help you lose weight in the short term. They can also be a major cause of the inflammatory changes in your gut-brain axis, which can cause damage to your body and the brain. It also means that you'd be smart to scan labels for artificial sweeteners, and avoid them whenever possible.

Food Emulsifiers

Emulsifiers are detergent-like molecules that help mix two liquids that don't easily mix, like oil and water. The food industry adds them routinely to a variety of foods, including mayonnaise, sauces, candy, and a range of bakery products, in order to create a uniform consistency. You can recognize them by their chemical names on food labels, such as sorbitan trisearate in chocolate, polysorbates in ice cream, and citric acid esters in processed meat, to name just a few. But these detergent-like molecules come with a downside. They can disrupt the protective mucus layer that covers the inner surface of the gastrointestinal tract, giving gut microbes easier access to the gut lining. Food emulsifiers also can disrupt the tight seal formed by the intact intestinal lining, enabling gut bacteria to cross and gain access to nearby immune cells, promoting metabolic toxemia.

To find out whether gut microbes play a role in the detrimental effects of emulsifiers on the gut, Andrew Gewirtz's group at Emory University recently fed low concentrations of two commonly used food emulsifiers—polysorbate 80 and carboxymethylcellulose—to mice. This induced low-grade intestinal inflammation, obesity, and features of metabolic syndrome. The gut microbiota of these animals attached closer to the intestinal lining, the mix of microbes in the gut changed, and LPS levels increased, just as they do in animals fed a high-fat diet.

Emulsifiers did not cause these metabolic changes in mice that were fed antibiotics, suggesting that gut microbiota played a key role. The investigators further confirmed this when they transplanted stool from the emulsifier-treated mice to germ-free mice and saw the same metabolic changes.

Besides the dangers of commonly used food additives for our metabolic health, there are major implications for the functioning of our gut-microbiome-brain axis and our brain health. From these experiments, it's clear that food emulsifiers, just as animal fat and artificial sweeteners, can change the profile of your gut microbiota in a way that is conducive to the development of low-grade inflammation in your gut, other organs, and in the brain, including the appetite-control regions of your brain. Too much of these ingredients and you might be prone to overeating high-calorie foods, which would only aggravate the inflammation and make the situation worse. Unfortunately, there is more to be concerned about in our diet that may affect brain health.

Vital Gluten

Take a walk down the aisles of any high-end grocery store and you'll see gluten-free breads, gluten-free pasta, gluten-free cereal, even gluten-free soft drinks or wine. Over the past decade, the so-called gluten-free diet has skyrocketed in popularity. Today, according to one recent survey, up to one-third of all adult Americans consume gluten-free products in any given year.

Gluten is a mix of proteins that makes up 12 to 14 percent of the protein content in wheat, and it's also found, to a lesser extent, in barley and rye, and in products made from any of these grains. Wheat is the most widely grown crop worldwide, and wheat flour, of course, is used to make breads, pastas, bagels, pizza, cereal, and many other common food items. Gluten is everywhere in the North American diet.

Gluten is also purified from wheat to create a food additive known as "vital gluten." Food manufacturers add vital gluten to a wide variety of foods, including bread, breakfast cereal, and even meat products. Vital gluten adds many qualities to foods, including an optimal texture and chewiness of bread, as well as an extended shelf life. It also helps to bind water and fats in processed meats. Vital gluten is being added to foods that have some gluten naturally (breads, pasta, pizza, beer) and those that don't, including meat products, sauces, and milk—amazingly enough—even nonfood products and cosmetics. The average American's gluten intake from flour and grains has increased more than 30 percent in the past half century, from 9 pounds per year in 1970 to 12 pounds per year in 2000, while the consumption of gluten additives mixed into various foods has increased at least threefold.

Should you even worry about all this extra gluten?

You definitely should if you're among the 1 percent of the population that has celiac disease, which causes the immune system to overreact to gluten and produce antibodies to the lining of the intestine. These antibodies remain in the body, producing chronic symptoms, including abdominal pain, diarrhea, weight loss, fatigue, and in severe cases neurological symptoms—and some of the symptoms can remain even after the patient stops eating wheat.

Celiac disease has been on the rise for sixty years, and now it affects 1 percent of people worldwide. No one knows exactly why. One proposed hypothesis is the increased consumption of gluten-containing foods; another is a change in the immune system, possibly related to the alterations in the way the gut-based immune system is trained early on in life by interacting with foreign microorganisms. A third hypothesis is related to alterations in how wheat has been modified and is grown.

You should also be careful if you're among the small minority of the population with a wheat allergy, in which the immune system produces an allergy-causing antibody called immunoglobulin E, or IgE, to gluten and other wheat proteins. Eating wheat can be serious, even life-threatening if you have wheat allergy, causing hives, nasal congestion, abdominal cramps, and a swollen mouth or throat that can make it hard to swallow or breathe.

A gluten-free diet will typically help alleviate symptoms in both of the above, well-established conditions. The widespread availability of gluten-free products is an enormous help for such individuals to lead lives without debilitating symptoms.

But if you don't have any of these symptoms, should you worry about what vital gluten in foods is doing to your brain? Despite recent widespread claims that gluten is harmful to every human being, there is currently no good scientific evidence to support this extreme view. I have yet to meet a French or Italian person who would give up the consumption of delicious fresh-baked crispy baguettes, the soft and moist ciabatta bread, or the savory pasta dishes for the uncertain benefits of freeing themselves from common ailments that have existed since long before the recent surge in vital gluten.

Linda Schmidt was convinced that her symptoms must be related to gluten sensitivity. A middle-aged woman, Schmidt would eat gluten-containing grains, then hours or days later suffer from a variety of symptoms resembling irritable bowel syndrome: sensations of bloating, gurgling in her belly, visible abdominal distension, abdominal pain and discomfort, irregular bowel habits, fatigue, and brain fog. Her gastroenterologist had done a comprehensive diagnostic evaluation and ruled out celiac disease. Nevertheless, after reading about gluten sensitivity and hearing discussions about it in the media, Linda had embarked on a gluten-free diet. According to Linda, the results were remarkable: Soon after she made the switch, she said, her digestive symptoms improved, her brain fog lifted, and she felt generally better than she had for a long time.

I see patients like Linda Schmidt regularly. They do not have a diagnosis of celiac disease, yet they report dramatic improvement of their IBS symptoms once they switch to a gluten-free diet (though they still come to see me with their residual symptoms).

It's possible that popular books and media attention to gluten sensitivity, and the promise of a miracle cure for common bothersome gastrointestinal and often associated symptoms of fatigue, loss of energy, and chronic pain, have lured many to a gluten-free diet. We may even be witnessing a mass hysteria around gluten-containing foods, one that's fanned by the marketing campaigns of a multibillion-dollar gluten-free-food industry.

But it's also possible that the North American diet is doing something to our brain-gut-microbiome axis, and that Linda Schmidt may have a third type of gluten-related disorder called nonceliac gluten sensitivity, a condition that appears to be much more common than celiac disease but remains poorly understood. Currently available science on this condition is sketchy at best. Small studies have shown that people with nonceliac gluten sensitivity do not have abnormal immune reactions and their guts are not leaky, as one might have expected from listening to proponents of the gluten hypersensitivity concept. Could it be that the increased amounts of vital gluten act through gut microbes to produce metabolites that are bad for our well-being? Or could it be that rather than gluten itself, it is the processed foods with all their other additives, most of which are also high in vital gluten, that are the main culprits?

The definitive answer to these questions are not yet in, and it may take science a while to provide it. Believers in the evils of dietary gluten do not need such scientific confirmation of what they are convinced is a well-established disorder. High fat content, artificial sweeteners, food emulsifiers, and other factors in our diet may have altered the set point of the myriad of sensors within our gut, including many of the receptors on nerve endings, enteroendocrine cells, and immune cells. Remember, the gut is our most complex sensory organ. Such changes may have altered the signals our gut sends to the enteric nervous system and to our brain. Is it possible that people with the most sensitive guts—people like Linda Schmidt—are now showing signs of food sensitivities and food allergies that they might not previously have developed? They may just be the canaries in the coal mine, experiencing problems long before the rest of us notice.

How the North American Diet May Contribute to Chronic Diseases of the Brain

Aubrey's constipation had developed gradually over two years, and by the time he arrived at my clinic, his symptoms were so severe that he needed daily laxatives and lots of straining to have regular bowel movements. As I took his history, Aubrey, who was fifty-five, told me that unless he took those measures, he might not have a bowel movement for several days.

I listened for clues as to what might be causing Aubrey's

symptoms. He was not taking a medication that causes constipation as a side effect, such as calcium channel blockers that patients take for high blood pressure. And he was not in the early stages of depression, which can bring on constipation. When I asked Aubrey about his dietary habits, there was nothing unusual. He had been eating a typical North American diet for all his life, his favorite foods being steaks, hot dogs, and hamburgers. I wasn't sure at first what was causing his symptoms, but when I happened to glance at his hands, I noticed a very slight tremor of his right index finger and thumb.

Tremors like this can be an early symptom of Parkinson's disease, which afflicts more than 7 million people worldwide, including 1 million Americans. The classic symptoms of advanced Parkinson's are familiar to many: characteristic hand tremors, slow movement, rigid or stiff muscles, impaired posture and balance. These symptoms reflect degeneration in several brain regions that contain dopamine as a neurotransmitter, which are involved in motor coordination. But long before these classical neurological symptoms appear, patients often develop GI symptoms. Such symptoms, particularly constipation, affect up to 80 percent of Parkinson's patients, and they can precede the onset of the classical neurological symptoms by decades.

It has long been known that nerve cells in affected brain regions contain so-called Lewy bodies—abnormal clumps of protein that interfere with nerve function. As the earliest symptoms of constipation develop in the gut, is it possible that Parkinson's disease begins in the gut and gradually makes its way to the brain? Could Parkinson's disease be a gut-brain disorder? And could the gut's microbiome be one of the culprits? Based on exciting new scientific evidence, the answer to all these questions may be yes.

It turns out that the protein that clumps to form Lewy bodies, alpha-synuclein, exists not only in patients' brains, but also in nerve cells within their gut. In fact, certain nerve cells in the enteric nervous system degenerate years before other Parkinson's symptoms appear, compromising the elaborate functioning of the little brain in the gut, slowing peristalsis, and delaying the transit of stool through the colon. It has been proposed that a person might eat food or drink water containing a neurotropic virus—a virus that preferentially infects nerve cells—which would gradually make its way through the lining of the intestine into the enteric nervous system. From there it could move inexorably up the vagus nerve—the information superhighway that is so essential to transmit gut sensations to the brain. From the vagus nerve it could infect the brain stem and move to brain regions controlling movement and mood.

While no such virus has been identified to date, researchers have identified changes in patients' gut microbiota that could make such an infection process easier, or that could promote the growth of such viruses normally living in the gut. Gut microbiota undergo major shifts in Parkinson's patients, as demonstrated in a recent study performed by Filip Scheperjans, of the University of Helsinki, and his colleagues. The investigators found that the microbiota of Parkinson's patients had reduced levels of Prevotella bacteria compared with the microbiota of healthy people. Perhaps not coincidentally, Prevotella flourish in the guts of people who eat a plant-based diet, and are reduced in people who eat fewer plants and more meat, milk, and dairy. We don't know if these gut microbial changes in patients with Parkinson's disease play any causative role in the disease, or if they are a consequence of the altered gut environment associated with Parkinson's. And they may only become important when other factors are in place, such as genetic vulnerability or other environmental toxins. Many parts of the Parkinson's disease puzzle are still missing. But other types of studies also offer supporting evidence that Parkinson's, too, might be a disease of the brain-gut-microbiome axis. A vegetarian diet, which shifts the microbiome, lowers the risk of Parkinson's disease, for example. And we know gut microbial diversity wanes later in life, a period when your gut microbiome becomes more vulnerable to disturbances. Perhaps not coincidentally, Parkinson's usually sets in after the age of sixty.

If this hypothesis pans out, then early dietary interventions to calm the gut's immune system might help prevent the onset of Parkinson's disease in high-risk patients, or at least slow its progression. And shifting away from the typical North American diet may help many people to prevent the onset of Parkinson's.

Rediscovering the Mediterranean Diet

Two years ago, I had the pleasure of visiting my friend Marco Cavalieri and his lovely wife, Antonella, who own an organic winery in the town of Fermo, a small town in the Marche region of Italy, just south of Ancona on the Adriatic coast. It's a land of rolling hills covered with small patches of bright yellow sunflowers, vineyards, olive trees, and wheat fields that slope gently to the blue sea. Patches of different plants and crops are often separated by rows of trees, bushes, and cornflowers, creating an unintended design masterpiece that embodies themes of beauty, harmony, and connectedness. The visual appeal of the scenery is a reflection of an incredible diversity of plants used in agriculture. When we arrived at nine thirty in the evening, we expected only that we would share a light dinner with our friends. Instead our hosts welcomed us at a restaurant close to the Piazza del Popolo. Fully consistent with its name, which means Place of the People, the piazza was filled with groups of townspeople engaged in conversations and children playing soccer. After we were greeted by the restaurant owner, a friend of the Cavalieris, a series of small, delicious dishes appeared on our table in sequence: whole-grain lasagna as an appetizer, brisket goose, seasonal roasted vegetables, chicory, grilled octopus, pecorino cheese, and local olives. All the dishes were prepared with local olive oil, some of it pressed from olives growing on the same ancient trees that the Benedictine monks had planted eight hundred years ago! There was not a trace of animal fat in anything we consumed. By the end of the evening we had also finished two bottles of organically grown wine from Marco's vineyards.

As families strolled up and down the piazza, Marco explained some of the unique aspects of how people in this area of Italy grew, harvested, and consumed their food and wine. The majority of foods people eat originate less than fifty miles away—from the fresh fish caught in the Adriatic to the many types of regional cheeses, the olives and fresh fruit, and the wild boars and deer hunted in the fall. The geographically restricted food supply meant there was a strong seasonal pattern to the types of meals that were prepared, based on the availability of local food ingredients. The emphasis on diverse regional products extended to the local wines: different grapes were grown in soils of different chemical composition in areas that varied in their closeness to the sea and the amount of sunshine they received.

Fermo is clearly a spiritual place, and not just because it has produced four popes—statues of whom decorate each side of the piazza. Its history of agriculture dates back to A.D. 890, when the Benedictine monks came to the area and established the monastery of Farfa. For four hundred years the Farfensi monks contributed to the great prosperity of the region, largely through their farming and their teaching of farming. Following their belief in the concept of *Ora et labora* (pray and work), they worked the land, studied, and wrote down their insights.

Many of these handwritten volumes can still be viewed in the old library adjacent to the piazza.

The first bottle of wine we had with the lasagna was a dry, white wine made exclusively from the pecorino grape. Marco explained that the grape's name comes from its use by the shepherds in the mountains, who also made the pecorino cheese that we enjoyed with the wine. He also pointed out how the logo of his winery depicts a monk picking a bunch of grapes so tenderly that it's almost a caress. Marco emphasized that this same passion, attention, and respect for nature and its products lives on in the Cavalieris' vineyard, which is named after the Benedictine monks: "Le Corti Dei Farfensi."

By the time we got to the second bottle—an aged red wine made from a blend of Montepulciano and Sangiovese grapes from the southern Marche region—and finished our educational meal with a small serving of tiramisu, I'd learned volumes about the ancient and unique methods by which food and wine are produced in this part of the world. Most important, I'd come to realize that there is much more to Mediterranean cuisine than a list of major food components and a meal's relative amounts of plant- and animal-based products. What we experienced firsthand in our few days of living in this environment showed that the close interdependence of historical, spiritual, environmental, and biological factors contributes significantly to the impressive health benefits of the Mediterranean diet.

In a pleasant departure from the world of ever-changing fad diets, there is a remarkable consensus among nutrition experts regarding the health benefits of the Mediterranean diet and closely related diets. Traditional Mediterranean diets have evolved over two thousand years, starting when the ancient Greeks and Romans dominated the area, with later input from African and Arab countries bordering the Mediterranean Sea. These different influences have yielded a remarkably high diversity of fruits and other plant-based foods that are cultivated, processed, and consumed in various region-specific dishes in countries bordering the sea. A typical Mediterranean diet contains at least 5 servings of vegetables, 1–2 servings of legumes and beans, 3 servings of fruit, 3–5 servings of grains, 5 servings of plant fats (olive oil, avocado, nuts, and seeds), consumption of seafood 2–4 times per week, and red meat not more than 1 time per week. The health benefits of the Mediterranean diet were first systematically studied in the 1950s and 1960s during the Seven Countries Study, a research project lead by Mayo Clinic investigator Ancel Keys that included subjects from the town of Montegiorgio, which is also in the Marche region of Italy, where Marco grows his organic grapes and olives. Although the specifics of the diet vary depending on the country and region, and even though there have been significant changes in the dietary habits since the time of the initial study, the basic dietary pattern is characterized by high consumption of monounsaturated fatty acids—primarily from olive oil—as well as daily consumption of fruits, vegetables, whole-grain cereals, low-fat dairy products, and moderate amounts of red wine; weekly consumption of fish, poultry, nuts, and legumes; and low and infrequent consumption of red meat. While the average fat content of the Mediterranean diet can range from 20 percent in Sicily to 35 percent in Greece, the great majority of this fat comes from plant sources, in particular olive oil. There is an extensive medical literature based on epidemiological studies and clinical trials that document the beneficial role of the Mediterranean diet with regard to mortality from all causes, particularly metabolic syndrome, cardiovascular disease, cancer, cognitive impairment, and depression. The health benefits were recently confirmed in a large study that combined all the previously published literature, covering more than half a million people.

The evidence in favor of the Mediterranean diet for brain health is not limited to large epidemiological studies. A recent study performed in nearly seven hundred elderly adults living in the U.S., all of whom underwent brain imaging studies to identify possible correlations between the brain and the Mediterranean diet, demonstrated larger volumes in many brain regions in subjects strictly adhering to a Mediterranean diet compared to those who did less so. Lower consumption of meat and higher consumption of fish were the main factors explaining these differences. In another study, investigators assessed dietary habits in 146 elderly individuals and studied their brains nine years later. On the basis of dietary assessment, 26 percent of participants had a low Mediterranean diet score, indicating poor adherence to the diet; 47 percent had medium scores, and 27 percent had higher scores, representing the best adherence to the diet. The investigators found a strong association between adherence to the Mediterranean diet and brain imaging measures related to the integrity of nerve brain tissue in the bundles connecting different brain regions.

Several mechanisms have been proposed to explain the extensive health benefits of the Mediterranean diet. Besides the high levels of protective antioxidants and polyphenols contained in olive oil and red wine, which have beneficial effects on cellular health, the anti-inflammatory effect of the Mediterranean diet on the body is most often cited. Polyphenols are plant-based compounds found in a variety of foods and beverages. Besides red grapes and olives, many other fruits and vegetables are rich sources of polyphenols, as are coffee, tea, chocolate, and some nuts.

On a recent October day, I rejoined Marco out in the hills to watch the annual olive harvest. On a particular day, when about 30 percent of the olives on the trees have ripened, a massive effort is launched to harvest the fruit and get it to the processing plant within hours of the harvest. Marco's workers harvest olives from about 1,800 trees in the surroundings of Fermo, the majority of which are between five hundred and eight hundred years old! Not only was the age of these trees impressive—their size was as well. It would take two people to stretch their arms around their twisted trunks, and their roots extend up to one hundred feet in all directions, sampling nutrients from a large area of fertile soil that is teeming with microbe-producing nutrients. All the efforts of the harvest ritual—the age of the trees, picking of the mostly green olives, immediate processing in a cold press facility—are aimed to preserve the maximum amount of polyphenol content.

Based on scientific analyses that Marco performs on the fresh-pressed olive oil every year, it is obvious that the polyphenol content in oil made from these ancient olive trees is several-fold higher than that from younger trees, where most of the commercially available oil comes from. I wondered about the reason underlying the relationship of the age of the tree with the polyphenol content. Could it be that the trees produce their own longevity cocktail, in the form of chemical compounds that keep them healthy, productive, and resilient against disease and climate fluctuations? Is there a relationship between the number of healthy and active people in their nineties whom we saw walking in this area (confirmed by several scientific surveys), the age and health of this remarkable trees, and the regular consumption of this medicinal olive oil?

The Mediterranean diet features the same high ratio of plant-derived food products to animal-based foods contained in the prehistoric diets of the Yanomamis and Hazdas, as well as some of today's niche diets, including pescatarians and vegetarians. We now know that, in addition to the high levels of complex carbohydrates in this largely plant-based diet, it is the high levels of polyphenols that exert a beneficial effect on the gut microbiota. The polyphenols not only come from the daily consumption of extra virgin olive oil; these health-promoting compounds are also contained in nuts, berries, and red wine, all of which are essential elements of the Mediterranean diet. A recent small study has even demonstrated that red wine ingestion may have a favorable influence on our gut microbiota composition.

While I have been focusing on the traditional Mediterranean diet as an example for the health benefits of a largely plant-based diet, there are other traditional dietary habits around the world which have demonstrated similar positive effects on health. They include the traditional Japanese diet, including the Okinawan diet, and the traditional Chinese and Korean diets. Even though these diets have evolved in different parts of the world, in different climate zones, in people from different races, they all are deeply embedded in the respective culture and belief systems, sometimes even tied to religious traditions. Not surprisingly, all these health promoting diets share the high ratio of plant- to animal-derived food items associated with high dietary fiber consumption, and the high intake of products with anti-inflammatory and disease fighting molecules. A rapidly evolving body of scientific evidence is now showing us the crucial role that our gut microbiome plays in translating these diets into health of body and brain.

Despite all of the research proving the remarkable benefits of these health-promoting diets, we should always be careful not to forget the aspects of diet less easily measured by science. The feeling of social connectedness when sharing a delicious meal and the attitude and outlook of those enjoying can't be empirically assessed. But a close look at the rituals and social interactions associated with the consumption of food in different parts of Asia or the experiences I had when visting Fermo is any indication, these factors engaging the entire mind-gut microbiome axis likely play an important role.

CHAPTER 10

THE SIMPLE ROAD
TOWARD WELLNESS AND
OPTIMAL HEALTH

‖‖

The intense information exchange between your brain, your gut, and its microbiota takes place twenty-four hours a day, regardless if you sleep or are awake, from the day you are born to the day you die. All of that communication isn't just coordinating your basic digestive functions—it also impacts our human experience, including how we feel, how we make decisions, how we socialize, and how much we eat. And if we listen carefully, this conversation can also guide us toward optimal health.

We are living in unprecedented times. What we eat and drink has changed dramatically, and we are exposed to more chemicals and drugs than any people who ever lived. We are beginning to learn how these changes, along with chronic life stress, can affect not only the gut microbes, but also their complex dialogue with the gut and the brain. These conversations play an important, well-established role in common syndromes of the gastrointestinal tract, in particular IBS, as well as in some forms of obesity. And we are beginning to recognize how disturbances in the gut microbial world can influence our brain. Recent studies have implicated altered brain-gut-microbiota interactions in brain disorders such as depression, anxiety, autism, Parkinson's, and even Alzheimer's disease. But even those of us who don't suffer from these diseases can improve our health by learning more about this vital conversation.

What Is Optimal Health?

A couple of years ago, a longtime friend of mine, Melvin Schapiro, was traveling with his wife and two other couples from San Juan, Puerto Rico, heading for a vacation on a remote island in the Caribbean. Mel and his friends had done the trip many times in the past; however, on this occasion something went awfully wrong. The small propeller plane that was carrying them had inadvertently been fueled with jet fuel and shortly after takeoff it crashed. Mel and his fellow travelers miraculously survived, some with serious injuries requiring hospitalization. Mel sustained several fractured ribs and a broken vertebra as well as a deep gash in his lower leg that required minor surgery at the local trauma center. Within hours of the injury he was flown back to Los Angeles for hospitalization and further medical care. Now here comes the most remarkable part of the story: despite these traumatic and emotional injuries, he was soon walking with crutches and just three weeks after the accident was working in his office and preparing for an important medical conference only a month away.

Only a small percentage of people in the United States live in a state of optimal health, a condition that has been defined

THE SIMPLE ROAD TOWARD WELLNESS AND OPTIMAL HEALTH   265

as complete physical, mental, emotional, spiritual, and social well-being, with peak vitality, optimal personal performance, and high productivity. In other words, it's a person who not only has no bothersome physical symptoms but is also happy, optimistic, has lots of friends, and enjoys his or her work. My friend Mel is such a unique individual. Every once in a while, we read about these people in the news, people like Fauja Singh, the so-called Turbaned Tornado, who began running at eighty-nine and completed the London marathon at 101. "Life is a waste without humor—living is all about happiness and laughter," Singh says.

Several colleagues of mine in their late seventies and even eighties remain fully active, healthy, and highly productive, pursuing their research, teaching students, seeing patients, conducting large international studies, and traveling around the world talking about their work at scientific meetings. If there is one personal characteristic that stands out among all of them, it is their curiosity and excitement about all things in life, their positive view of the world, and their unwillingness to be bogged down by negative people or events. Their gut-based decisions seem to have a consistently positive bias, assuming that no matter what, they will be okay. It is also not uncommon to hear stories of a remarkable ability to bounce back from health issues—such as my friend's plane crash— or personal losses such as the death of a spouse. All these individuals seem to have a high degree of resilience—an ability to return to a healthy steady state after unanticipated events in life have thrown them off balance.

It has been estimated that superhealthy people make up less than 5 percent of the North American population. Optimal health has been a popular topic in the lay media, but it is not a goal that physicians are trained to help their patients achieve. Traditionally, a large part of our health care system—a more appropriate name for it would be our disease care system—has focused almost exclusively on treating the symptoms of chronic disease, maximizing its efforts on expensive screening diagnostics and equally expensive long-term pharmacological treatments. Similarly, federally funded biomedical research is almost exclusively focused on unraveling disease mechanisms and not on identifying the biological and environmental factors that contribute to a state of optimal health.

Much more common than the superhealthy are people like Sandy, a highly successful, middle-aged, divorced professional living on the West Side of Los Angeles. Sandy had been struggling to meet her professional obligations and be a good mother to her two teenage daughters. Although she had a sensitive stomach for as long as she could remember, she, like the majority of people with such mild sensitivities, always considered herself healthy and had never consulted a physician for her symptoms. But she had noticed that she was getting tired more easily, didn't have as much energy as she used to, woke up in the morning feeling tired, and had gained fifteen pounds over the past year. She flew to the East Coast several times a month, often on a red-eye, and she had noticed that it took her longer to recover from the trip than in the past.

Sandy hadn't spent much time thinking about her digestive system until recently, except when she listened to the ubiquitous television commercials talking about beneficial effects of probiotic yogurts for digestive wellness, or the talk-show guests discussing the dangerous effects of gluten. She had read about the health benefits of a gluten-free diet for a wide range of symptoms similar to hers, and she was interested in getting my advice on how to optimize her gut microbiome through simple, specific dietary interventions.

Sandy is one of the large and growing proportion of the population who live in a state of suboptimal health you could call a "predisease" state. These people have received no official medical diagnosis. Their blood tests have turned up no biochemical evidence suggesting early disease. But they are likely to feel chronically stressed and worried, and it takes them longer to return to a relaxed state after a stressful experience. They are also more likely to be overweight or obese, have borderline elevated blood pressure, experience low-grade chronic digestive discomfort (ranging from heartburn to bloating and irregular bowel habits), and have limited time and energy for a fulfilling social life. They often experience poor sleep, loss of energy, symptoms of fatigue, and recurrent aches and pains in their bodies, in particular low back pain and headaches. They may also consider these symptoms as the price they have to pay for making a living for their family, or for a career in the fast lane. Even though such individuals often don't meet the diagnostic criteria doctors use to make a specific medical diagnosis, such as IBS, fibromyalgia, chronic fatigue syndrome, or mild hypertension, it is possible to identify several characteristic abnormalities on specialized tests, including markers of systemic inflammation in their bodies.

Such predisease states can be viewed as the consequences of the wear and tear on the body (the so-called allostatic load), which increases over time when a person experiences repeated minor stressors or is under constant, chronic stress. Many of us live in such a stressful world, but the wear and tear is harder on some individuals than on others. Repeated or prolonged activation of the stress circuits in the brain harms our metabolic, cardiovascular, and brain health. Allostatic load also has a major impact on our brain-gut-microbiome axis, presumably because our gut reactions affect gut microbial behavior. As the allostatic load increases, our gut microbes and their connection to the brain play a major role in mediating systemic inflammation. As inflammation worsens, levels of inflammatory markers in the bloodstream rise, including LPS, adipokines (signaling molecules produced by fat cells), and a substance called C-reactive protein.

As we have learned, diet can interact with our gut microbiota to cause similar inflammatory states, a situation called "metabolic toxemia." There is good reason to believe that several decades of metabolic toxemia in an otherwise healthy individual is enough to cause profound structural and functional changes to the brain.

Even more worrisome, gut reactions from chronic stress and a high-fat diet can combine to exacerbate the inflammatory state. They do so by increasing the gut's leakiness, making the gut microbiota more likely to activate the gut's immune system. High stress levels also drive many people toward the temptation of comfort foods, which then can make up-regulated stress circuits in the brain the new normal, which in turn further exacerbates inflammation in the gut in a vicious cycle.

The combination of feeding our gut microbes a diet high in animal fat, and the chronic wear and tear on our brain associated with chronic stress, represents the perfect storm to push us at some point—likely triggered by other, yet unknown factors—from the predisease state into such common health problems as metabolic syndrome, coronary vascular disease, cancer, and degenerative brain diseases.

Was I able to give Sandy sound medical advice, and answer her question about how to develop a healthy gut microbiome? And was I able to advise her how to move from the focus on her predisease state toward a goal of optimal health? The answer is yes. I strongly believe that everybody is able to work toward optimal health by focusing on establishing and maintaining balance within their gut-microbiome-brain axis. How? By maximizing its resilience.

What Is a Healthy Gut Microbiome?

To keep our gut microbiomes healthy, we first need to know what constitutes a healthy gut microbiome.

Since your gut microbiome is an ecosystem, it's helpful to think of it as an ecologist would. Think of the human body as a landscape, with different parts of the body as distinct zones, each of which provides its own distinct habitat for microorganisms. These range from the vagina, home to just a few species, to the mouth, which houses a diverse array of microbes. Even within the digestive system, there are distinct zones, including low-diversity habitats in the stomach and small intestine, and high-diversity habitats in our large intestine, which has more microbes than any other location in the body, and the largest diversity of microbes as well.

When I asked Daniel Blumstein, an ecologist and UCLA colleague, to describe a healthy ecological state, he reminded me that in natural habitats there can be several stable healthy states. In other words, all ecosystems display multiple stable states. In the case of the human microbial ecosystem, some stable states are associated with health, and others with disease.

To visualize the concept of stable states within an ecological system, I like to think about one of my favorite drives in California. Driving from Santa Barbara to Monterey on California's Highway 1, also known as the Pacific Coast Highway, I enjoy watching the golden, rolling hills covered with oak trees and vineyards give way to taller mountains divided by valleys as you get closer to the coast. Multiple factors have shaped this beautiful landscape, including the geology, rivers, earthquakes, tectonic shifts, weather, and the animals that have lived on it for thousands of years. Imagine if you could drop a giant ball onto this landscape from high in the air and watch it roll. You could easily predict that it would come to rest in the valleys and other depressions. The deeper these depressions are, the more effort it would then take to roll the ball over a hill into another valley. In other words, when the ball is in one of these depressions, it is in a stable state, and the deeper the depression, the more stable that state is.

By analogy, you can represent the microbial ecology of the gut as an equally hilly landscape on a three-dimensional graph. In this case, the distance from a depression to a hilltop represents how much energy it takes to roll the ball up the hill to get over to the next depression—which is what it takes to switch from one temporarily stable state to another. David Relman, a pediatrician and leading microbiologist from Stanford University, says the most stable microbial states in the gut— the valleys and most pronounced depressions—reflect states either of optimal health or chronic disease.

Many factors determine the landscape of your gut microbiome, analogous to the factors that have shaped natural landscapes. One important factor is your genetic makeup and the way these genes are modified through the influence of early life experiences, good and bad. The activity of your immune system is also important, as are your eating habits, lifestyle, and environment and the nature of your unique gut reactions, which reflect your habits of mind.

A limited number of longitudinal studies have been completed on the composition of the gut microbiota, and they seem to show that dietary changes, immune function, and the use of medications, in particular antibiotics, can trigger shifts from one state to another. These shifts can be temporary, rapidly switching back to the healthy default state, or persistent, resulting in chronic disease. So depending on your gut microbial landscape, you may be more prone to develop prolonged digestive discomfort following a gut infection or show unhealthy

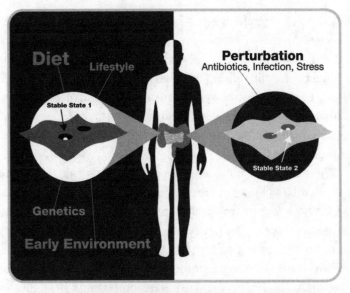

**FIG. 7. HOW ANTIBIOTICS, STRESS, AND INFECTIONS CAN CHANGE THE
ECOLOGICAL LANDSCAPE OF THE GUT MICROBIOME**

*Using terminology from ecology, the gut organization and
function of the gut microbiome can best be conceptualized as a
stability landscape with hills and valleys; the deeper the valleys,
the more resistant the state is to perturbations. The stability of
the state is determined by a variety of factors including genes and
early life events. When the system is perturbed sufficiently, it will
leave its original stable state and move to a new state, which can
be stable or transient. Many of these new states are associated
with disease. The most common perturbations are antibiotics,
infections, or stress.*

spikes in blood sugar following a dessert. This microbial landscape may determine who will benefit more from switching to
a healthy diet or from taking probiotics, and who will be more
sensitive to the effects of a course of antibiotics.

Diversity. One of the generally agreed-upon criteria for a healthy gut microbiome has been its diversity and the abundance of microbial species present in it. As in the natural ecosystems around us, high diversity of the microbiome means resilience and low diversity means vulnerability to perturbations. Fewer microbial species means a diminished ability to withstand perturbations such as infections (by pathogenic bacteria, viruses, or the pathobionts living in our gut), poor diet, or medications.

There are some noticeable exceptions to this rule, including the microbiota living in the gut of a newborn and in the vagina, which have low microbial diversity when they're healthy, and for good reasons. The newborn's microbiome needs flexibility in order to create a pattern of communities of gut microbes during the early programming period, which is unique for each individual. The vaginal microbiome needs flexibility in order to adjust its function to the unique demands of reproduction and delivery. Nature has developed clever alternative strategies to ensure the stability of these unique habitats and protect them from infections and disease. Both habitats are dominated by lactobacilli and bifidobacteria. These bacteria can produce many antimicrobial substances, and they have the unique ability to produce enough lactic acid to create an acidic milieu that is hostile to most other microorganisms and pathogens.

Someone with low-diversity, relatively unstable gut microbial communities may never show any signs of overt disease. However, when the microbiota of such high-risk individuals are perturbed, diseases are more likely to develop. A growing scientific literature demonstrates that diseases such as obesity, inflammatory bowel disease, and other autoimmune disorders are associated with reduced gut microbial diversity, often as a consequence of repeated exposure to antibiotics. Other diseases may join this list in the future.

Unfortunately, it seems easier to reduce gut microbial diversity in an adult than to increase it above the level of diversity established during the first three years of life. For example, it is relatively easy to decrease gut microbial diversity at any age by taking antibiotics, but studies suggest it's difficult to increase our normal level of microbial diversity, thereby increasing our resilience against disease and improving our health. No matter how many probiotic pills you swallow, how much sauerkraut and kimchi you consume, and how extreme a diet you select, your basic gut microbial composition and diversity will remain relatively stable.

That's no reason to throw up your hands, however. We know that probiotic interventions can benefit your gut health by altering the metabolites that your microbiota produce. The impact of such a probiotic intervention on the health of your gut microbes may be greater during the first few years in life, when the microbiome is still developing, or following the decimation of your gut microbial diversity from intake of a broad-spectrum antibiotic, or during chronic life stress.

How does gut microbial diversity protect against disease? Diversity is closely linked to two critical properties of healthy ecosystems—stability and resilience.

Stability and resilience. Although you may carry different microbial species than your coworker or cousin, you tend to carry the same key set of species for long periods. This stability is critical for your health and well-being. It ensures that friendly gut microbes can return quickly to an equilibrium state following a stress-related perturbation, which allows them to keep up their beneficial activities over time. This makes a microbiome resilient.

Conversely, some people's gut microbiota are especially sensitive to perturbation. Mrs. Stone, who developed protracted symptoms of a gastroenteritis during her vacation in Mexico, clearly started out with a gut microbiome that was less resilient and stable than that of her fellow vacationers. Was her microbial landscape altered by the chronic stress she was under at the time of her vacation? Or did she start out with a less stable microbial landscape from the first years of her life, when a series of early adverse life events permanently changed it?

The emerging ecological view of gut microbial health contrasts with claims promoted by the food supplement industry and by the media that a healthy microbiome is composed of defined populations of specific species of microbes. In fact, only 10 percent of gut microbial species are shared between individuals. In other words, you and a friend might both have a healthy microbiome, but you might have vastly different communities of gut microbes. Put another way, there are several stable healthy states of the gut microbiota.

All this means that no quick analysis of your gut bacterial species—for example, your ratio of Prevotella to Bacteroides, or Firmicutes to Bacteroidetes—can assess the integrity of your gut-brain axis and your health status. It also means that it's really not possible to provide a one-size-fits-all recommendation about which probiotics to take or which dietary intervention will provide specific benefits.

Vastly different communities of gut microbes, however, can produce very similar patterns of metabolites. This suggests that future tests will assess gut microbiome health not simply by looking for specific microbial populations, but by looking at which genes are expressed and which metabolic pathways are active.

We cannot expect that any simple intervention by itself, such as a particular diet, will optimize your gut microbiome, while not paying attention to all the other factors that influence gut microbial function, like the influence of unhealthy gut reactions associated with stress, anger, and anxiety at the same time. Nor will simply eating your daily probiotic-enriched yogurt while continuing your high-animal-fat, low-plant-food diet, trying out kimchi or sauerkraut for a short period of time, or eliminating grains, complex carbohydrates, or gluten from your diet. None of these interventions by themselves will improve a chronically disturbed dialogue between the gut and the brain. Switching to a gluten-free diet even though you have no evidence for celiac disease will make the billion-dollar gluten-free industry happy, but in most cases it will not have any long-lasting effect on your own well-being and health. The science now says that changing your diet is not enough. You need to modify your lifestyle as well.

When Is the Time to Invest in Optimal Health?

The brain-gut-microbiome axis is most vulnerable to health-harming perturbations during three periods: from pregnancy through infancy (the perinatal period), adulthood, and old age. And scientists now agree that the first few years in life, starting during development in the womb, matter most for our long-term health and well-being.

Our gut-microbiota-brain interactions are shaped early in life, from before birth to age eighteen, through our interactions with the world—our psychosocial influences, diet, and chemicals in our food (including antibiotics, food additives, artificial sweeteners, and more). Early life—from before birth to age three—is a particularly crucial period for the shaping of the gut microbial architecture. Both the microbiome and brain circuits are still developing, and changes during this time tend to persist for life. Furthermore, gut sensations and associated emotional feelings are being filed into the database in your

brain, shaping for life your background emotions, tempera-
ment, and ability to make beneficial gut decisions.

Throughout adult life, both what we eat and how we feel exert a profound influence on the chemical conversations our gut
microbes have with other key players in our intestine, including immune cells, hormone- and serotonin-containing cells,
sensory nerve endings, and more. This "gut-based caucus"
sends signals back to the brain, influencing our desire to eat,
our stress sensitivity, how we feel, and how we make our gut
decisions. Meanwhile, our emotions, and their associated gut
reactions, exert a profound influence on the complex dialogue
in our gut, and this exerts a large influence on what type of
messages the gut sends back to the brain.

The consequences of altering the gut-microbiota-brain dialogue may not manifest until later in life, when the diversity
and resilience of the gut microbiota both decrease. This makes
it likely to make us more vulnerable to developing degenerative
brain disorders such as Alzheimer's or Parkinson's disease. To
prevent these devastating disorders, we need to pay attention
to how we treat our gut-brain-microbiota axis much earlier in
life, long before the damage of the brain manifests as serious
symptoms.

Improving Your Health by Targeting
the Gut Microbiome

As we rapidly untangle the complex chemical conversations between microbes, the gut, and the nervous system, we're also
extracting valuable information about how to apply this knowledge to improve people's health.

But before we can offer evidence-based recommendations,

we have important research questions to answer. David Relman, the Stanford University microbiology expert, has recently summarized them: What are the most important processes and factors that determine human microbiota assembly after birth? Does the mix of gut microbes as a child alter your risk of health and disease as an adult? What are the most important determinants of microbiome stability and resilience? How can you make your gut microbiota more stable and resilient, and how can you restore it to health when it's not? To answer these and other questions, we need carefully designed clinical studies that assess multiple, possibly interacting disease factors, including the microbiome.

Down the road, if we could assess a person's gut microbial landscape and signaling molecules generated in this system, we could determine his or her vulnerability to antibiotics, stress, diet, and other destabilizing factors and design personalized treatments that could prevent the development of diseases, or restore the gut microbiome to health—through lifestyle modifications, dietary interventions, or future medical therapies. A recent study demonstrated that customized dietary recommendations improved blood sugar control following a meal, based on multiple personal factors, including the gut microbiome configuration.

We might also be able to spot early warning signs in the microbiome of future diseases of the body or the brain. A gut microbial analysis from a simple stool sample could become one of the most powerful screening tools in health care. This could help detect particular diseases, or vulnerability to particular diseases, including poorly understood brain-gut disorders such as autism spectrum disorders, Parkinson's disease, Alzheimer's disease, and depression.

Novel therapies are possible. Microbiologists and CEOs of start-up companies are busy mining the human gut microbiome for novel therapies, using new computational tools. They've already found a wealth of new drug candidates within the human microbiota. They also hope to patent genetically engineered probiotic microbes to treat various diseases, including anxiety, depression and brain-gut disorders like IBS or chronic constipation, by changing a patient's gut microbial architecture. But this may prove more difficult than they think. Microbiota consist of many interacting species, which makes it difficult to control, add, or target individual species without affecting the overall ecological balance. In the distant future, expensive new treatments that use nanotechnologies and genetically engineered probiotics to manipulate our own microbiota may be able to target individual microbes within a complex ecosystem, but for the foreseeable future, it may not be the practical way to go.

Instead, there are approaches that anyone can take today without spending a lot of money. In a recent *Science* article, Jonas Schluter and Kevin Foster, of the University of Oxford, propose that we act as "ecosystem engineers" and manipulate general, system-wide properties of microbial communities to our benefit. This implies that you have a basic understanding of the building plans of the system and should always be skeptical of simplistic solutions that are promoted with the promise to optimize your health.

How can we do this?

Practice natural and organic farming of your gut microbiome. Consider your gut microbiome as a farm and your microbiota as your own personal farm animals, then decide what to feed them to optimize their diversity, stability, and health, and optimize production of beneficial signaling molecules that affect our brains. Would you feed them food items that you knew were loaded with potentially harmful chemicals or enriched with unhealthy additives? This will be the first step in taking control of what you eat. It will increase your awareness next time you go to the market, are tempted to buy fast food for lunch, or debate whether you should order a dessert.

Cut down on animal fat in your diet. All the animal fat in the typical North American diet, regardless if it is visible or hidden in many processed foods, is bad for your health. It plays a major role in increasing your waistline, and recent data has shown that processed meat, which has a particularly high fat content, enhances your risk of developing several types of malignancies, including cancers of the breast, colon, and prostate. High animal fat intake is also bad for your brain health. There is growing evidence that dietary fat–induced changes in gut microbial signaling to the brain via the gut's immune system can change our nervous system both functionally and structurally. Since our brain-gut axis has not evolved to cope with a daily avalanche of fat and corn syrup, and a high-fat diet sets up a vicious cycle of dysregulated eating behavior that harms your brain health, become aware of these unhealthy consequences.

Maximize your gut microbial diversity. If you want to maximize your gut microbial diversity, increase its resilience, and reduce your vulnerability to chronic diseases of the brain, follow the old advice of nutritionists, cardiologists, and public health officials: in addition to eating moderate quantities of meats low in fat, mainly from fish and poultry, increase your intake of food items that contain multiple prebiotics in the form of different plant fibers, a combination of food items that we know today leads to greater gut microbial diversity.

Indigenous people living in the Amazonian rain forest know hundreds of dietary and medicinal plants, and eat a large variety of wild animal products. Over hundreds of thousands of years, our gut sensory mechanisms have evolved to recognize and encode a large number of such nutritional and medicinal plant signals. There are an impressive number of gut sensors that respond to a wide variety of herbs and phytochemicals, from wasabi to hot peppers, from mint to sweet and bitter tastes, to name just a few. We know that signals from these herbs and foods are transmitted to the brain and the enteric nervous system and that they have an important effect both on our digestion and on the way we feel. Nature would not have come up with these mechanisms over millions of years of evolution unless they provided a health benefit.

Learn to listen to your gut, which in this context means to remember that your gut has evolved an elaborate system to handle a huge variety of naturally grown vegetables, fruits, and other plant-derived foods, as well as smaller amounts of animal protein, but that it struggles to handle all the fat, sugar, and additives that the food industry adds to processed foods. Unless you have been diagnosed with potentially serious medical disorders, such as a specific food allergy (such as seafood and peanut allergies) or celiac disease, try to avoid extreme diets that limit the natural variety of foods, in particular plant-based food items. Develop your own personalized diet within the general constraints of the "ground rules" of high-diversity foods, mainly from plant sources.

Avoid mass-produced and processed foods and maximize organically grown food. Follow the advice that Michael Pollan gives in his recent book, *Food Rules*. Buy only things in the market that look like food. If they don't, they most likely will contain food additives that could harm your brain, including artificial sweeteners, emulsifiers, fructose corn syrup, and vital gluten, to name just a few. For the same reasons, watch out for the hidden dangers in food you buy in the supermarket. Read labels to find out the components and additives in a food item;

try to find out where it comes from. If you do this regularly, you will often be surprised that your fish or poultry comes from a country without rules for how these animals are raised and what they are fed, and how many calories are in a bag of so-called reduced-fat chips.

Modern food producers have abandoned any consideration of the complexity of the microbial world and the importance of natural diversity of life, choosing instead to maximize output and profitability. Industrial farming of beef, poultry, fish, and other seafood defies ecological principles, creating patches of devastated ecological landscapes sustainable only through the use of antibiotics and other chemicals. Furthermore, the waste produced by these livestock and fish farms, and the antibiotic-resistant microorganisms that escape them, harms surrounding habitats as well. Ultimately, products coming from such surrounding compromised ecosystems—be it the water, soil, or air—will find their way to you, and will be a risk for your health.

Reducing the microbial diversity in the soil, on plants, and in the GI tract of farm animals may ultimately harm our own gut microbiome and our nervous system. Keep in mind that pesticides used to grow GMO foods may not directly harm our human bodies, but they are likely to affect the function and health of our gut microbes and their interactions with the brain. The same holds true for residues of low-dose antibiotics that remain in many mass-produced meat and seafood products.

Eat fermented foods and probiotics. While the science is still evolving, it's still prudent to maximize your regular intake of fermented food products and all types of probiotics to maintain gut microbial diversity, especially during times of stress, antibiotic intake, and old age. All fermented foods contain probiotics—live microorganisms with potential health benefits, and a few commercially available probiotics contained in fermented milk products, drinks, or in pill form have been evaluated for their health benefits. Unfortunately, there are also hundreds of such products in all shapes and forms, whose producers make vague claims of health benefits. Yet for many of them, we don't even know if enough live organisms reach your small and large intestine to exert their claimed beneficial effects. But people have been eating naturally fermented, unpasteurized foods for thousands of years, and you might want to include some of them in your regular diet. Such products include kimchi, sauerkraut, kombucha, and miso, to name just a few. Various fermented milk products, including kefir, different types of yogurts, and hundreds of different cheeses, provide probiotics as well. I recommend selecting low-fat and low-sugar products that are free of emulsifiers, artificial coloring, and artificial sweeteners.

If you consume fermented dairy products, such as probiotic-enriched yogurts, you are also feeding your own microbes an important source of prebiotics (such as the milk oligosaccharides we discussed in the previous chapter), and if you're eating fermented vegetables, you're feeding your gut microbes another form of prebiotics, such as dietary fiber from complex plant carbohydrates. Probiotic bacteria you eat as an adult do not become a permanent part of your gut microbiota, but regular intake of probiotics may help to maintain gut microbial diversity during times of trouble, and it can normalize the pattern of metabolites produced by your gut microbes.

Be mindful of prenatal nutrition and stress. If you're a woman of reproductive age, it is equally important to remember that your diet will influence your child as well—from pregnancy, through childbirth and the period of breastfeeding, until the child is three years old, when his or her gut microbes are fully established. The maternal gut microbiome produces metabolites that can influence fetal brain development, and diet-induced inflammation of the gut-microbiome-brain axis may harm a fetus's developing brain. In fact, full-blown inflammation during pregnancy is a major risk factor for brain diseases such as autism and schizophrenia, and low-grade inflammation from a mother's high-fat diet may be sufficient to adversely affect the fetal brain development in more subtle ways. On the other hand, stress during pregnancy or maternal stress when the child grows up has well-documented negative effects on the development of the brain and the gut microbiota, often resulting in child behavioral problems.

Eat smaller portions. This limits the calories you consume, keeping the amount in line with your body's metabolic needs, and simultaneously reduces your fat intake. When eating packaged foods, be aware of the recommended serving size on the label. The calorie count on your potato chip bag may seem reasonable, but it refers to eating just a few chips. Eating the whole bag may serve up far more calories and fat than what you want to eat that day.

Fast to starve your gut microbes. Periodic fasting has been an integral part of many cultures, religions, and healing traditions for thousands of years, and prolonged fasting may have positive impact on brain functions and well-being. A popular explanation for the benefits of fasting is based on the idea that it cleanses the gut and the body by getting rid of harmful and toxic substances. Even though people have believed this throughout history, there is little scientific evidence for this hypothesis. But based on what we now know about brain-gut-microbiota interactions, fasting may have a profound effect on the composition and function of your gut microbiome and possibly on your brain.

Recall that when your stomach is empty, it activates periodic high-amplitude contractions that slowly but forcefully sweep from the esophagus to the end of the colon. At the same time, the pancreas and the gallbladder secretion release a synchronized burst of digestive juices. The combined effect of this reflex, called the migrating motor complex, is analogous to a weekly neighborhood street sweeping. We don't yet know what this street sweeping does to our gut microbes or whether it alters the metabolites they produce. There is good evidence that it removes microbes from the small intestine, where normally only a few reside, and sweeps them into the colon, where most gut microbes live. In people with an inactive migrating motor complex, microbes grow more abundantly in the interior of the small intestine, a condition called small intestinal bacterial overgrowth. This causes abdominal discomfort, bloating, and altered bowel habits. We don't know whether fasting also reduces the abundance of microbes living in the large intestine, and if the microbes living in close proximity to the lining of the gut are affected as well.

Fasting may also reset the many sensory mechanisms in the gut that are essential for gut-brain communication. These include our main appetite control mechanisms, which sense satiety. Having no fat in the intestine for one or more days may enable vagal nerve endings to regain their sensitivity to appetite-reducing hormones such as cholecystokinin or leptin, and it may also return sensitivity settings in the hypothalamus to normal levels.

Don't eat when you are stressed, angry, or sad. To farm your gut microbes optimally, feeding is only half the story. We've seen that emotions can have a profound effect on the gut and the microbial environment in the form of gut reactions. A negative emotional state will throw the gut-microbiota-brain axis out of balance in several ways. It makes your gut leakier, it activates your gut-based immune system, and it triggers endocrine cells in the gut wall to release signaling molecules such as the stress hormone norepinephrine and serotonin. It can also reduce important members of your gut microbial communities, in particular lactobacilli and bifidobacteria. These can profoundly change the behavior of gut microbes. These behavioral changes are likely to influence the structure of microbial communities, how the microbes break down food components, and which metabolites they send back to the brain.

For all these reasons, no matter how conscientious you are when selecting your food at the Whole Foods market, and no matter how much you believe in the health benefits of the latest fad diet, feelings of stress, anger, sadness, or anxiety always turn up at your dinner table. They can not only ruin the meal; if you eat when you're feeling bad, it can also be bad for your gut and bad for your brain. Think about Frank, who became intolerant to food when worried about not being close enough to a restroom in an unfamiliar restaurant, or Bill, who couldn't stop vomiting when he was stressed. If you are not mindful of the stress or other negative emotions in your body, it can lead you into seeking comfort food, even though such food is unhealthy.

For these reasons, scan your body and mind and tune in to your emotions before you sit down to eat something. If you are stressed, anxious, or angry, try to avoid adding food to the turmoil in your gut.

In addition, if you have always been an anxious person, or suffer from an anxiety disorder or depression, the influence of these negative mind states on the activities of your gut microbes when it comes to digesting the leftovers of your meal is even more pronounced, and it may be difficult to change the situation even if you are aware of it. In this case, it is prudent to seek the help of a physician or psychiatrist to treat such common conditions.

Enjoy meals together. Just as negative emotions are bad for your gut-microbe-brain axis, happiness, joy, and a feeling of connectedness are probably good. If you eat when you're happy, your brain sends signals to your gut that you can think of as special ingredients that spice up your meal and please your microbes. I suspect that happy microbes will in turn produce a different set of metabolites that benefit your brain. As noted by the authors of several scientific articles about the Mediterranean diet, some of the health benefits you get from eating a Mediterranean diet are likely to come from the close social interactions and lifestyle common in countries adhering to such a diet. The resulting sense of connectedness and well-being almost certainly affects the gut and influences how your gut microbiota respond to what you eat.

After scanning your body and becoming aware of how you feel, try to switch to a positive emotional state and experience the difference this shift has on your overall well-being. Various techniques have been proven effective at this, including cognitive behavioral therapy, hypnosis, and self-relaxation techniques, as well as mindfulness-based stress reduction. You may see benefits every time you eat a meal, or you may notice benefits that occur over time.

Become an Expert in Listening to Your Gut Feelings

Mindfulness-based stress reduction can also help you get in touch with your gut feelings and reduce the negative biasing influence of thoughts and memories on these feeling states. This sort of mindfulness helps relieve disorders of the gut-brain axis.

Mindfulness meditation is typically described as "nonjudgmental attention to experiences in the present moment." In order to become more mindful you will have to master three interrelated skills: learn to focus and sustain your attention in the present moment, improve your ability to regulate your emotions, and develop a greater self-awareness. Under normal circumstances, the majority of bodily signals reaching your brain are not consciously perceived. A key element of mindfulness meditation is learning to become more aware of these bodily sensations, including the sensations associated with deep abdominal breathing, and with the state of your digestive system. By becoming more aware of these gut feelings, those associated with good and bad gut reactions, you can better regulate your own emotions. According to brain-imaging studies, including those performed by my colleague Kirsten Tillisch, meditation affects key brain regions that help you pay attention and make value judgments about the world around you and about events going on in your body. It also leads to structural changes in several brain regions, including those involved with body awareness, memory, regulation of emotions, and anatomical connections between the right and left hemisphere.

Keep Your Brain (and Your Gut Microbiota) Fit

Of course, there is unequivocal evidence for the health-promoting effects of regular exercise, and no recommendations to achieve optimal health could come without the inclusion of regular physical exercise. Aerobic exercise has well-documented beneficial effects on brain structure and function, ranging from a reduction in the age-related decline in thickness of the cerebral cortex, to improved cognitive function and reduced stress responsiveness. In view of the close interactions between the brain, the gut, and its microbes, there is no question in my mind that these brain-related health benefits of regular exercise are reflected in a positive way in the health of the gut microbiome.

HOW AND WHAT TO FEED YOUR GUT MICROBES

- Aim to maximize gut microbial diversity by maximizing regular intake of naturally fermented foods and probiotics.

- Reduce the inflammatory potential of your gut microbiota by making better nutritional choices.

  - Cut down on animal fat in your diet.

  - Avoid, whenever possible, mass-produced, processed food and select organically grown food.

- Eat smaller servings at meals.

- Be mindful of prenatal nutrition.

- Reduce stress and practice mindfulness.

- Avoid eating when you are stressed, angry, or sad.

- Enjoy the secret pleasures and social aspects of food.

- Become an expert in listening to your gut feelings.

Even though we humans are fascinated by the exploration of the frontiers in space and in the vastness of the oceans, it seems that until recently, we completely ignored the complex universe within our own bodies. While much is still to be learned about the influence of this system on our health and well-being, the emerging science is already having a major influence on our mind and body.

The brain-gut-microbiome axis links our brain health closely to what we eat, how we grow and process our food, what medications we take, how we come into this world, and how we interact with the microbes in our environment throughout life. Now that we are beginning to fully understand this marvelous complexity of universal connectedness, in which we as humans represent only a tiny fraction, I am convinced that we will view the world, ourselves, and our health with very different eyes.

This new awareness will shift our focus from treating diseases toward achieving optimal health. It will shift us away from spending billions on treating cancer with warlike, scorched-earth therapies, on treating obesity with crippling surgeries of the gastrointestinal tract, and on dealing with the fallouts from cognitive decline with expensive long-term support measures. It will shift us away from being passive recipients of an ever-increasing number of medications to taking responsibility for the optimal functioning of our brain-gut axis by becoming ecological systems engineers with the knowledge, power, and motivation to get our gut-microbiota-brain interactions functioning at peak effectiveness, with the goal of optimal health.

ACKNOWLEDGMENTS

I have benefited from the contribution of many individuals who have made it possible to write this book. I am grateful to my patients who over several decades have taught me with their life stories the importance of mind-brain-gut interactions for health and disease. To my incredible colleagues and research team who were essential throughout my career in pursuing the research on the interactions between the gut, its microbiota, and the brain. To Paul Bell, Sue Smalley, and Barb Natterson, who encouraged me to embark on writing this book and whose encouragement helped me to complete it. To Rob Lemelson and Marco Cavalieri, who with their incredible generosity provided beautiful physical spaces to start the creative writing process. To Dan Ferber for invaluable advice and assistance that helped me to put a wealth of hard science into an easily readable and entertaining text, and to Sandra Blakesley, Billi Gordon, and Royce Flippin for their creative input. To Mark Lyte for help with historical aspects of the gut-microbiome signaling story. To Marco Cavalieri and Nancee Chaffee for practical advice on the topic of the Mediteranean diet. To Catherine Cowles, my agent, who introduced me to the world of publishing for a wide audience and to Julie Will, my editor at HarperWave, who put her faith into my book proposal from the very beginning and provided me invaluable editorial advice throughout the process. To Jon Lee, for creating the illustrations for the book. And last but not least to my wife, Minou, who not only encouraged me to keep on going during difficult phases of the writing process, but who was incredibly supportive by putting up with an "absent" husband during the past year.

BIBLIOGRAPHY

Aagaard, Kjersti, Jun Ma, Kathleen M. Antony, Radhika Ganu, Joseph Petrosino, and James Versalovic. "The Placenta Harbors a Unique Microbiome." *Science Translational Medicine* 6 (2014): 237ra65.

Abell, Thomas L., Kathleen A. Adams, Richard. G. Boles, Athos Bousvaros, S. K. F. Chong, David R. Fleisher, William L. Hasler, et al. "Cyclic Vomiting Syndrome in Adults." *Neurogastroenterology and Motility* 20 (2008): 269–84.

Aksenov, Pavel. "Stanislav Petrovic: The Man Who May Have Saved the World." BBC News, September 26, 2013. http://www.bbc.com/news/world-europe-24280831.

Albenberg, Lindsey G., and Gary D. Wu. "Diet and the Intestinal Microbiome: Associations, Functions, and Implications for Health and Disease." *Gastroenterology* 146 (2014): 1564–72.

Alcock, Joe, Carlo C. Maley, and C. Athena Aktipis. "Is Eating Behavior Manipulated by the Gastrointestinal Microbiota? Evolutionary Pressures and Potential Mechanisms." *Bioessays* 36 (2014): 940–49.

Allman, John M., Karli K. Watson, Nicole A. Tetreault, and Atiya Y. Hakeem. "Intuition and Autism: A Possible Role for Von Economo Neurons." *Trends in Cognitive Neurosciences* 9 (2005): 367–73.

Almy, Thomas P., and Maurice Tulin. "Alterations in Colonic Function in Man Under Stress. I. Experimental Production of Changes Simulating the Irritable Colon." *Gastroenterology* 8 (1947): 616–26.

Aziz, Imran, Marios Hadjivassiliou, and David S. Sanders. "The Spectrum of Noncoeliac Gluten Sensitivity." *Nature Reviews Gastroenterology and Hepatology* 12 (2015): 516–26.

Baeckhed, Fredrik, Josefine Roswall, Yangqing Peng, Qiang Feng, Huijue Jia, Petia Kovatcheva-Datchary, Yin Li, et al. "Dynamics and Stabilization of the Human Gut Microbiome During the First Year of Life." *Cell Host and Microbe* 17 (2015): 690–703.

Bailey, Michael T., Gabriele R. Lubach, and Christopher L. Coe. "Prenatal Stress Alters Bacterial Colonization of the Gut in Infant Monkeys." *Journal of Pediatric Gastroenterology and Nutrition* 38 (2004): 414–21.

Bailey, Michael T., Scot E. Dowd, Jeffrey D. Galley, Amy R. Hufnagle, Rebecca G. Allen, and Mark Lyte. "Exposure to a Social Stressor Alters the Structure of the Intestinal Microbiota: Implications for Stressor-Induced Immunomodulation." *Brain, Behavior and Immunity* 25 (2011): 397–407.

Bercik, Premysl, Emmanuel Denou, Josh Collins, Wendy Jackson, Jun Lu, Jennifer Jury, Yikang Deng, et al. "The Intestinal Microbiota Affect Central Levels of Brain-Derived Neurotropic Factor and Behavior in Mice." *Gastroenterology* 141 (2011): 599–609, 609.e1–3.

Berdoy, Manuel, Joanne P. Webster, and David W. Macdonald. "Fatal Attraction in Rats Infected with Toxoplasma gondii." *Proceedings of the Royal Society B: Biological Sciences* 267 (2000): 1591–94.

Bested, Alison C., Alan C. Logan, and Eva M. Selhub. "Intestinal Microbiota, Probiotics and Mental Health: From Metchnikoff to Modern Advances: Part II—Contemporary Contextual Research." *Gut Pathogens* 5 (2013): 3.

Binder, Elisabeth B., and Charles B. Nemeroff. "The CRF System, Stress, Depression, and Anxiety: Insights from Human Genetic Studies." *Molecular Psychiatry* 15 (2010): 574–88.

Blaser, Martin. *Missing Microbes*. New York: Henry Holt, 2014.

Braak, Heiko, U. Rüb, W. P. Gai, and Kelly Del Tredici. "Idiopathic Parkinson's Disease: Possible Routes by Which Vulnerable Neuronal Types May Be Subject to Neuroinvasion by an Unknown Pathogen." *Journal of Neural Transmission (Vienna)* 110 (2003): 517–36.

Bravo, Javier A., Paul Forsythe, Marianne V. Chew, Emily Escaravage, Hélène M. Savignac, Timothy G. Dinan, John Bienenstock, and John F. Cryan. "Ingestion of Lactobacillus Strain Regulates Emotional Behavior and Central GABA Receptor Expression in a Mouse via the Vagus Nerve." *Proceedings of the National Academy of Sciences USA* 108 (2011): 16050–55.

Bronson, Stephanie L., and Tracy L. Bale. "The Placenta as a Mediator of Stress Effects on Neurodevelopmental Reprogramming." *Neuropsychopharmacology* 41 (2016): 207–18.

Buchsbaum, Monte S., Erin A. Hazlett, Joseph Wu, and William E. Bunney Jr. "Positron Emission Tomography with Deoxyglucose-F18 Imaging of Sleep." *Neuropsychopharmacology* 25, no. 5 Suppl (2001): S50–S56.

Caldji, Christian, Ian C. Hellstrom, Tie-Yuan Zhang, Josie Diorio, and Michael J. Meaney. "Environmental Regulation of the Neural Epigenome." *FEBS Letters* 585 (2011): 2049–58.

Cani, Patrice D., and Amandine Everard. "Talking Microbes: When Gut Bacteria Interact with Diet and Host Organs." *Molecular Nutrition and Food Research* 60 (2016): 58–66.

Champagne, Frances, and Michael J. Meaney. "Like Mother, like Daughter: Evidence for Non-Genomic Transmission of Parental Behavior and Stress Responsivity." *Progress in Brain Research* 133 (2001): 287–302.

Chassaing, Benoit, Jesse D. Aitken, Andrew T. Gewirtz, and Matam Vijay-Kumar. "Gut Microbiota Drives Metabolic Disease in Immunologically Altered Mice." *Advances in Immunology* 116 (2012): 93–112.

Chassaing, Benoit, Omry Koren, Julia K. Goodrich, Angela C. Poole, Shanthi Srinivasan, Ruth E. Ley, and Andrew T. Gewirtz. "Dietary Emulsifiers Impact the Mouse Gut Microbiota Promoting Colitis and Metabolic Syndrome." *Nature* 519 (2015): 92–96.

Chu, Hiutung, and Sarkis K. Mazmanian. "Innate Immune Recognition of the Microbiota Promotes Host-Microbial Symbiosis." *Nature Immunology* 14 (2013): 668–75.

Collins, Stephen M., Michael Surette, and Premysl Bercik. "The Interplay Between the Intestinal Microbiota and the Brain." *Nature Reviews Microbiology* 10 (2012): 735–42.

Costello, Elizabeth K., Keaton Stagaman, Les Dethlefsen, Brendan J. M. Bohannan, and David A. Relman. "The Application of Ecological Theory Toward an Understanding of the Human Microbiome." *Science* 336 (2012): 1255–62.

Coutinho, Santosh V., Paul M. Plotsky, Marc Sablad, John C. Miller, H. Zhou, Alfred I. Bayati, James A. McRoberts, and Emeran A. Mayer. "Neonatal Maternal Separation Alters Stress-Induced Responses to Viscerosomatic Nociceptive Stimuli in Rat." *American Journal of Physiology—Gastrointestinal and Liver Physiology* 282 (2002): G307–16.

Cox, Laura M., Shingo Yamanashi, Jiho Sohn, Alexander V. Alekseyenko, Jacqueline M. Young, Ilseung Cho, Sungheon Kim, Hullin Li, Zhan Gao, Douglas Mahana, Jorge G. Zarate Rodriguez, Arlin B. Rogers, Nicolas Robine, P'ng Loke, and Martin Blaser. *Cell* 158 (2014): 705–721.

Coyte, Katherine Z., Jonas Schluter, and Kevin R. Foster. "The Ecology of the Microbiome: Networks, Competition, and Stability." *Science* 350 (2015): 663–66.

Craig, A. D. How *Do You Feel? An Interoceptive Moment with Your Neurobiological Self*. Princeton, NJ: Princeton University Press, 2015.

———. "How Do You Feel—Now? The Anterior Insula and Human Awareness." *Nature Reviews Neuroscience* 10 (2009): 59–70.

———. "Interoception and Emotion: A Neuroanatomical Perspective." In *Handbook of Emotions*, 3rd ed. Edited by Michael Lewis, Jeannette M. Haviland-Jones, and Lisa Feldman Barrett, 272–88. New York: Guilford Press, 2008.

Critchley, Hugo D., Stefan Wiens, Pia Rotshtein, Arne Öhman, and Raymond J. Dolan. "Neural Systems Supporting Interoceptive Awareness." *Nature Neuroscience* 7 (2004): 189–95.

Cryan, John F., and Timothy G. Dinan. "Mind-Altering Microorganisms: The Impact of the Gut Microbiota on Brain and Behaviour." *Nature Reviews Neuroscience* 13 (2012): 701–12.

Damasio, Antonio. *Descartes' Error: Emotion, Reason, and the Human Brain*. New York: Putnam, 1996.

———. *The Feeling of What Happens: Body and Emotion in the Making of Consciousness*. New York: Harcourt Brace, 1999.

Damasio, Antonio, and Gil B. Carvalho. "The Nature of Feelings: Evolutionary and Neurobiological Origins." *Nature Reviews Neuroscience* 14 (2013): 143–52.

David, Lawrence A., Corinne F. Maurice, Rachel N. Carmody, David B. Gootenberg, Julie E. Button, Benjamin E. Wolfe, Alisha V. Ling, et al. "Diet Rapidly and Reproducibly Alters the Human Gut Microbiome." *Nature* 505 (2014): 559–63.

De Lartigue, Guillaume, Claire Barbier de La Serre, and Helen E Raybould. "Vagal Afferent Neurons in High Gat Diet-Induced Obesity: Intestinal Microflora, Gut Inflammation and Cholecystokinin." *Physiology and Behavior* 105 (2011): 100–105.

De Palma, Giada, Patricia Blennerhassett, J. Lu, Y. Deng, A. J. Park, W. Green, E. Denou, et al. "Microbiota and Host Determinants of Behavioural Phenotype in Maternally Separated Mice." *Nature Communications* 6 (2015): 7735.

Diaz-Heijtz, Rochellys, Shugui Wang, Farhana Anuar, Yu Qian, Britta Björkholm, Annika Samuelsson, Martin L. Hibberd, Hans Forssberg, and Sven Petterssonc. "Normal Gut Microbiota Modulates Brain Development and Behavior." *Proceedings of the National Academy of Sciences USA* 108 (2011): 3047–52.

Dinan, Timothy G., and John F. Cryan. "Melancholic Microbes: A Link Between Gut Microbiota and Depression?" *Neurogastroenterology and Motility* 25 (2013): 713–19.

Dinan, Timothy G., Catherine Stanton, and John F. Cryan. "Psychobiotics: A Novel Class of Psychotropic." *Biological Psychiatry* 74 (2013): 720–26.

Dorrestein, Pieter C., Sarkis K. Mazmanian, and Rob Knight. "Finding the Missing Links Among Metabolites, Microbes, and the Host." *Immunity* 40 (2014): 824–32.

Ernst, Edzard. "Colonic Irrigation and the Theory of Autointoxication: A Triumph of Ignorance over Science." *Journal of Clinical Gastroenterology* 24 (1997): 196–98.

Fasano, Alessio, Anna Sapone, Victor Zevallos, and Detlef Schuppan. "Nonceliac Gluten Sensitivity." *Gastroenterology* 148 (2015): 1195–1204.

Flint, Harry J., Karen P. Scott, Petra Louis, and Sylvia H. Duncan. "The Role of the Gut Microbiota in Nutrition and Health." *Nature Reviews Gastroenterology and Hepatology* 9 (2012): 577–89.

Francis, Darlene D., and Michael J. Meaney. "Maternal Care and the Development of the Stress Response." *Current Opinion in Neurobiology* 9 (1999): 128–34.

Furness, John B. "The Enteric Nervous System and Neurogastroenterology." *Nature Reviews Gastroenterology and Hepatology* 9 (2012): 286–94.

Furness, John B., Brid P. Callaghan, Leni R. Rivera, and Hyun-Jung Cho. "The Enteric Nervous System and Gastrointestinal Innervation: Integrated Local and Central Control." *Advances in Experimental Medicine and Biology* 817 (2014): 39–71.

Furness, John B., Leni R. Rivera, Hyun-Jung Cho, David M. Bravo, and Brid Callaghan. "The Gut as a Sensory Organ." *Nature Reviews Gastroenterology and Hepatology* 10 (2013): 729–40.

Gershon, Michael D. "5-Hydroxytryptamine (Serotonin) in the Gastrointestinal Tract." *Current Opinion in Endocrinology, Diabetes and Obesity* 20 (2013): 14–21.

———. *The Second Brain.* New York: HarperCollins, 1998.

Groelund, Minna-Maija, Olli-Pekka Lehtonen, Erkki Eerola, and Pentti Kero. "Fecal Microflora in Healthy Infants Born by Different Methods of Delivery: Permanent Changes in Intestinal Flora after Cesarean Delivery." *Journal of Pediatric Gastroenterology and Nutrition* 28 (1999): 19–25.

Grupe, Dan W., and Jack B. Nitschke. "Uncertainty and Anticipation in Anxiety: An Integrated Neurobiological and Psychological Perspective." *Nature Reviews Neuroscience* 14 (2013): 488–501.

Gu, Yian, Adam M. Brickman, Yaakov Stern, Christina G. Habeck, Qolamreza R. Razlighi, Jose A. Luchsinger, Jennifer J. Manly, Nicole Schupf, Richard Mayeux, and Nikolaos Scarmeas. "Mediterranean Diet and Brain Structure in a Multiethnic Elderly Cohort." *Neurology* 85 (2015): 1744–51.

Hamilton, M. Kristina, Gaëlle Boudry, Danielle G. Lemay, and Helen E. Raybould. "Changes in Intestinal Barrier Function and Gut Microbiota in High-Fat Diet-Fed Rats Are Dynamic and Region Dependent." *American Journal of Physiology—Gastrointestinal and Liver Physiology* 308 (2015): G840–51.

Henry J. Kaiser Family Foundation. "Health Care Costs: A Primer. How Much Does the US Spend on Health Care and How Has It Changed." May 1, 2012. http: //kff.org/report-section/health-care-costs-a-primer-2012-report/.

———. "Snapshots: Health Care Spending in the United States and Selected OECD Countries." April 12, 2011. http://kff.org/health-costs/

issue-brief/snapshots-health-care-spending-in-the-united-states-selected-oecd-countries/.

Hibbelna, Joseph R., Kate Northstone, Jonathan Evans, and Jean Golding. "Vegetarian Diets and Depressive Symptoms Among Men." *Journal of Affective Disorders* 225 (2018): 13–17.

Hildebrandt, Marie A., Christian Hoffman, Scott A. Sherrill-Mix, Sue A. Keilbaugh, Micah Hamady, Ying-Yu Chen, Rob Knight, Rexford S. Ahima, Frederic Bushman, and Gary D. Wul. "High-Fat Diet Determines the Composition of the Murine Gut Microbiome Independently of Obesity." *Gastroenterology* 137 (2009): 1716–24.e1–2.

House, Patrick K., Ajai Vyas, and Robert Sapolsky. "Predator Cat Odors Activate Sexual Arousal Pathways in Brains of Toxoplasma gondii Infected Rats." *PLoS One* 6 (2011): e23277.

Hsiao, Elaine Y. "Gastrointestinal Issues in Autism Spectrum Disorder." *Harvard Review of Psychiatry* 22 (2014): 104–11.

Human Microbiome Consortium. "A Framework for Human Microbiome Research." *Nature* 486 (2012): 215–21.

Iwatsuki, Ken, R. Ichikawa, A. Uematsu, A. Kitamura, H. Uneyama, and K. Torii. "Detecting Sweet and Umami Tastes in the Gastrointestinal Tract." *Acta Physiologica (Oxford)* 204 (2012): 169–77.

Jacka, Felice N., Adrienne O'Neil, Rachelle Opie, Catherine Itsiopoulos, Sue Cotton, Mohammedreza Mohebbi, David Castle, Sarah Dash, Cathrine Mihalopoulos, Mary Lou Chatterton, Laima Brazionis, Olivia M. Dean, Allison M. Hodge, and Michael Berk. "A Randomised Controlled Trial of Dietary Improvement for Adults with Major Depression (The 'SMILES' Trial)." *BioMed Central Medicine* 15 (2017) 23. doi: 10.1186/s12916-017-0791-y.

Jaenig, Wilfrid. *The Integrative Action of the Autonomic Nervous System: Neurobiology of Homeostasis.* Cambridge: Cambridge University Press, 2006.

Jasarevic, Eldin, Ali B. Rodgers, and Tracy L. Bale. "Alterations in the Vaginal Microbiome by Maternal Stress Are Associated with Metabolic Reprogramming of the Offspring Gut and Brain." *Endocrinology* 156 (2015): 3265–76.

———. "A Novel Role for Maternal Stress and Microbial Transmission in Early Life Programming and Neurodevelopment." *Neurobiology of Stress* 1 (2015): 81–88.

Jiang, Haiyin, Zongxin Ling, Yonghua Zhang, Hongjin Mao, Zhanping Ma, Yan Yin, Weihong Wang, Wenxin Tang, Zhonglin Tan, Jianfei Shi, Lanjuan Li, and Bing Ruan. "Altered Fecal Microbiota Composition in Patients with Major Depressive Disorder." *Brain, Behavior, and Immunity* 48 (2015): 186–194.

Johnson, Pieter T. J., Jacobus C. de Roode, and Andy Fenton. "Why Infectious Disease Research Needs Community Ecology." *Science* 349 (2015): 1259504.

Jouanna, Jacques. *Hippocrates*. Baltimore: Johns Hopkins University Press, 1999.

Karamanos, B., A. Thanopoulou, F. Angelico, S. Assaad-Khalil, A. Barbato, M. Del Ben, V. Dimitrijevic-Sreckovic, et al. "Nutritional Habits in the Mediterranean Basin: The Macronutrient Composition of Diet and Its Relation with the Traditional Mediterranean Diet: Multi-Centre Study of the Mediterranean Group for the Study of Diabetes (MGSD)." *European Journal of Clinical Nutrition* 56 (2002): 983–91.

Kastorini, Christina-Maria, Haralampos J. Milionis, Katherine Esposito, Dario Giugliano, John A. Goudevenos, and Demosthenes B. Panagiotakos. "The Effect of Mediterranean Diet on Metabolic Syndrome and Its Components: A Meta-Analysis of 50 Studies and 534,906 Individuals." *Journal of the American College of Cardiology* 57 (2011): 1299–1313.

Kelly, John R., Yuliya Borrea, Ciaran O' Brien, Elaine Patterson, Sahar El Aidy, Jennifer Deane, Paul J. Kennedy, Sasja Beers, Karen Scott, Gerard Moloney, Alan E. Hoban, Lucinda Scott, Patrick Fitzgerald, Paul Ross, Catherine Stanton, Gerard Clarke, John F. Cryan, and Timothy G. Dinan. "Transferring the Blues: Depression-Associated Gut Microbiota Induces Neurobehavioural Changes in the Rat." *Journal of Psychiatric Research* 82 (2016): 109–118.

Koenig, Jeremy E., Aymé Spor, Nicholas Scalfone, Ashwana D. Fricker, Jesse Stombaugh, Rob Knight, Largus T. Angenent, and Ruth E. Ley. "Succession of Microbial Consortia in the Developing Infant Gut Microbiome." *Proceedings of the National Academy of Sciences USA* 108 Suppl 1 (2011): 4578–85.

Krol, Kathleen M., Purva Rajhans, Manuela Missana, and Tobias Grossmann. "Duration of Exclusive Breastfeeding Is Associated with Differences in Infants' Brain Responses to Emotional Body Expressions." *Frontiers in Behavioral Neuroscience* 8 (2015): 459.

Le Doux, Joseph. *The Emotional Brain: The Mysterious Underpinnings of Emotional Life*. New York: Simon & Schuster, 1996.

Ley, Ruth E., Catherine A. Lozupone, Micah Hamady, Rob Knight, and Jeffrey I. Gordon. "Worlds Within Worlds: Evolution of the Vertebrate Gut Microbiota." *Nature Reviews Microbiology* 6 (2008): 776–88.

Lizot, Jacques. *Tales of the Yanomami: Daily Life in the Venezuelan Forest*. Cambridge: Cambridge University Press, 1991.

Lopez-Legarrea, Patricia, Nicholas Robert Fuller, Maria Angeles Zulet, Jose Alfredo Martinez, and Ian Douglas Caterson. "The Influence of Mediterranean, Carbohydrate and High Protein Diets on Gut Microbiota Composition in the Treatment of Obesity and Associated Inflammatory State." *Asia Pacific Journal of Clinical Nutrition* 23 (2014): 360–68.

Lyte, Mark. "The Effect of Stress on Microbial Growth." *Anima: Health Research Reviews* 15 (2014): 172–74.

Martin, Ioana A., Jennifer E. Goertz, Tiantian Ren, Stephen S. Rich, Suna Onengut-Gumuscu, Emily Farber, Martin Wu, Christopher C. Overall, Jonathan Kipnis, and Alban Gaultier. "Microbiota Alteration Is Associated with the Development of Stress-Induced Despair Behavior." *Nature Scientific Reports* (2017) 7:43859. DOI: 10.1038/srep43859.

Mawe, Gary M., and Jill M. Hoffman. "Serotonin Signaling in the Gut: Functions, Dysfunctions, and Therapeutic Targets." *Nature Reviews Gastroenterology and Hepatology* 10 (2013): 473–86.

Mayer, Emeran A. "Gut Feelings: The Emerging Biology of Gut-Brain Communication." *Nature Reviews Neuroscience* 12 (2011): 453–66.

———. "The Neurobiology of Stress and Gastrointestinal Disease." *Gut* 47 (2000): 861–69.

Mayer, Emeran A., and Pierre Baldi. "Can Regulatory Peptides Be Regarded as Words of a Biological Language." *American Journal of Physiology* 261 (1991): G171–84.

Mayer, Emeran A., Rob Knight, Sarkis K. Mazmanian, John F. Cryan, and Kirsten Tillisch. "Gut Microbes and the Brain: Paradigm Shift in Neuroscience." *Journal of Neuroscience* 34 (2014): 15490–6.

Mayer, Emeran A., Bruce D. Naliboff, Lin Chang, and Santosh V. Coutinho. "V. Stress and Irritable Bowel Syndrome." *American Journal of Physiology—Gastrointestinal and Liver Physiology* 280 (2001): G519–24.

Mayer, Emeran A., Bruce D. Naliboff, and A. D. Craig. "Neuroimaging of the Brain-Gut Axis: From Basic Understanding to Treatment of Functional GI disorders." *Gastroenterology* 131 (2006): 1925–42.

Mayer, Emeran A., David Padua, and Kirsten Tillisch. "Altered Brain-Gut Axis in Autism: Comorbidity or Causative Mechanisms?" *Bioessays* 36 (2014): 933–39.

Mayer, Emeran A., Kirsten Tillisch, and Arpana Gupta. "Gut/Brain Axis and the Microbiota." *Journal of Clinical Investigation* 125 (2015): 926–38.

McGovern Institute for Brain Research at MIT. "Brain Disorders by the Numbers." January 16, 2014. https: //mcgovern.mit.edu/brain-disorders/by-the-numbers#AD.

Menon, Vinod, and Luciana Q. Uddin. "Saliency, Switching, Attention and Control: A Network Model of Insula Function." *Brain Structure and Function* 214 (2010): 655–67.

Mente, Andrew, Lawrence de Koning, Harry S. Shannon, and Sonia S. Anand. "A Systematic Review of the Evidence Supporting a Causal Link Between Dietary Factors and Coronary Heart Disease." *Archives of Internal Medicine* 169 (2009): 659–69.

Moss, Michael. *Salt, Sugar, Fat.* New York: Random House, 2013.

Pacheco, Alline R., Daniela Barile, Mark A. Underwood, and David A. Mills. "The Impact of the Milk Glycobiome on the Neonate Gut Microbiota." *Annual Review of Animal Biosciences* 3 (2015): 419–45.

Panksepp, Jaak. *Affective Neuroscience. The Foundations of Human and Animal Emotions.* Oxford: Oxford University Press, 1998.

Pelletier, Amandine, Christine Barul, Catherine Féart, Catherine Helmer, Charlotte Bernard, Olivier Periot, Bixente Dilharreguy, et al. "Mediterranean Diet and Preserved Brain Structural Connectivity in Older Subjects." *Alzheimer's and Dementia* 11 (2015): 1023–31.

Pollan, Michael. *Food Rules: An Eater's Manual.* New York: Penguin Books, 2009.

Psaltopoulou, Theodora, Theodoros N. Sergentanis, Demosthenes B. Panagiotakos, Ioannis N. Sergentanis, Rena Kosti, and Nikolaos Scarmeas. "Mediterranean Diet, Stroke, Cognitive Impairment, and Depression: A Meta-Analysis." *Annals of Neurology* 74 (2013): 580–91.

Psichas, Arianna, Frank Reimann, and Fiona M. Gribble. "Gut Chemosensing Mechanisms." *Journal of Clinical Investigation* 125 (2015): 908–17.

Qin, Junjie, Ruiqiang Li, Jeroen Raes, Manimozhiyan Arumugam, Kristoffer Solvsten Burgdorf, Chaysavanh Manichanh, Trine Nielsen, et al. "A Human Gut Microbial Gene Catalogue Established by Metagenomic Sequencing." *Nature* 464 (2010): 59–65.

Queipo-Ortuno, Maria Isabel, María Boto-Ordóñez, Mora Murri, Juan Miguel Gomez-Zumaquero, Mercedes Clemente-Postigo, Ramon Estruch, Fernando Cardona Diaz, Cristina Andrés-Lacueva, and Francisco J. Tinahones. "Influence of Red Wine Polyphenols and Ethanol on the Gut Microbiota Ecology and Biochemical Biomarkers." *American Journal of Clinical Nutrition* 95 (2012): 1323–34.

Raybould, Helen E. "Gut Chemosensing: Interactions Between Gut Endocrine Cells and Visceral Afferents." *Autonomic Neuroscience* 153 (2010): 41–46.

Relman, David A. "The Human Microbiome and the Future Practice of Medicine." *Journal of the American Medical Association* 314 (2015): 1127–28.

Rook, Graham A., and Christopher A. Lowry. "The Hygiene Hypothesis and Psychiatric Disorders." *Trends in Immunology* 29 (2008): 150–58.

Rook, Graham A., Charles L. Raison, and Christopher A. Lowry. "Microbiota, Immunoregulatory Old Friends and Psychiatric Disorders." *Advances in Experimental Medicine and Biology* 817 (2014): 319–56.

Roth, Jesse, Derek LeRoith, E. S. Collier, N. R. Weaver, A. Watkinson, C. F. Cleland, and S. M. Glick. "Evolutionary Origins of Neuropeptides, Hormones, and Receptors: Possible Applications to Immunology." *Journal of Immunology* 135 Suppl (1985): 816s–819s.

Roth, Jesse, Derek LeRoith, Joseph Shiloach, James L. Rosenzweig, Maxine A. Lesniak, and Jana Havrankova. "The Evolutionary Origins of Hormones, Neurotransmitters, and Other Extracellular Chemical Messengers: Implications for Mammalian Biology." *New England Journal of Medicine* 306 (1982): 523–27.

Rutkow, Ira M. "Beaumont and St. Martin: A Blast from the Past." *Archives of Surgery* 133 (1998): 1259.

Sanchez, M. Mar, Charlotte O. Ladd, and Paul M. Plotsky. "Early Adverse Experience as a Developmental Risk Factor for Later Psychopathology: Evidence from Rodent and Primate Models." *Development and Psychopathology* 13 (2001): 419–49.

Sapolsky, Robert. "Bugs in the Brain." *Scientific American*, March 2003, 94.

Scheperjans, Filip, Velma Aho, Pedro A. B. Pereira, Kaisa Koskinen, Lars Paulin, Eero Pekkonen, Elena Haapaniemi, et al. "Gut Microbiota Are Related to Parkinson's Disease and Clinical Phenotype." *Movement Disorders* 30 (2015): 350–58.

Schnorr, Stephanie L., Marco Candela, Simone Rampelli, Manuela Centanni, Clarissa Consolandi, Giulia Basaglia, Silvia Turroni, et al. "Gut Microbiome of the Hadza Hunter-Gatherers." *Nature Communications* 5 (2014): 3654.

Schulze, Matthias B., Kurt Hoffmann, JoAnn E. Manson, Walter C. Willett, James B. Meigs, Cornelia Weikert, Christin Heidemann, Graham A. Colditz, and Frank B. Hu. "Dietary Pattern, Inflammation, and Incidence of Type 2 Diabetes in Women." *American Journal of Clinical Nutrition* 82 (2005): 675–84; quiz 714–15.

Seeley, William W., Vinod Menon, Alan F. Schatzberg, Jennifer Keller, Gary H. Glover, Heather Kenna, Allan L. Reiss, and Michael D. Greicius. "Dissociable Intrinsic Connectivity Networks for Salience Processing and Executive Control." *Journal of Neuroscience* 27 (2007): 2349–56.

Sender, Ron, Shai Fuchs, and Ron Milo. "Are We Really Vastly Outnumbered? Revisiting the Ratio of Bacterial to Host Cells in Humans." *Cell* 164 (2016): 337–340.

Shannon, Kathleen M., Ali Keshavarzian, Hemraj B. Dodiya, Shriram Jakate, and Jeffrey H. Kordower. "Is Alpha-Synuclein in the Colon a Biomarker for Premotor Parkinson's Disease? Evidence from 3 Cases." *Movement Disorders* 27 (2012): 716–19.

Smits, Samuel A., Jeff Leach, Erica D. Sonnenburg, Carlos G. Gonzalez, Joshua S. Lichtman, Gregor Reid, Rob Knight, Alphaxard Manjurano, John Changalucha, Joshua E. Elias, Maria Gloria Dominguez-Bello, and Justin L. Sonnenburg. "Seasonal Cycling in the Gut Microbiome of the Hadza Hunter-Gatherers of Tanzania." *Science* 357 (2017): 802–806.

Spiller, Robin, and Klara Garsed. "Postinfectious Irritable Bowel Syndrome." *Gastroenterology* 136 (2009): 1979–88.

Stengel, Andreas, and Yvette Taché. "Corticotropin-Releasing Factor Signaling and Visceral Response to Stress." *Experimental Biology and Medicine (Maywood)* 235 (2010): 1168–78.

Sternini, Catia, Laura Anselmi, and Enrique Rozengurt. "Enteroendocrine Cells: A Site of 'Taste' in Gastrointestinal Chemosensing." *Current Opinion in Endocrinology, Diabetes and Obesity* 15 (2008): 73–78.

Stilling, Roman M., Seth R. Bordenstein, Timothy G. Dinan, and John F. Cryan. "Friends with Social Benefits: Host-Microbe Interactions as a Driver of Brain Evolution and Development?" *Frontiers in Cellular and Infection Microbiology* 4 (2014): 147.

Sudo, Nobuyuki, Yoichi Chida, Yuji Aiba, Junko Sonoda, Naomi Oyama, Xiao-Nian Yu, Chiharu Kubo, and Yasuhiro Koga. "Postnatal Microbial Colonization Programs the Hypothalamic-Pituitary-Adrenal System for Stress Response in Mice." *Journal of Physiology* 558 (2004): 263–75.

Suez, Jotham, Tal Korem, David Zeevi, Gili Zilberman-Schapira, Christoph A. Thaiss, Ori Maza, David Israeli, et al. "Artificial Sweeteners Induce Glucose Intolerance by Altering the Gut Microbiota." *Nature* 514 (2014): 181–86.

Taché, Yvette. "Corticotrophin-Releasing Factor 1 Activation in the Central Amygdale and Visceral Hyperalgesia." *Neurogastroenterology and Motility* 27 (2015): 1–6.

Thaler, Joshua P., Chun-Xia Yi, Ellen A. Schur, Stephan J. Guyenet, Bang H. Hwang, Marcelo O. Dietrich, Xiaolin Zhao, et al. "Obesity Is Associated with Hypothalamic Injury in Rodents and Humans." *Journal of Clinical Investigation* 122 (2012): 153–62.

Tillisch, Kirsten, Jennifer Labus, Lisa Kilpatrick, Zhiguo Jiang, Jean Stains, Bahar Ebrat, Denis Guyonnet, Sophie Legrain-Raspaud, Beatrice Trotin, Bruce Naliboff, and Emeran A. Mayer. "Consumption of Fermented Milk Product with Probiotic Modulates Brain Activity." *Gastroenterology* 144 (2013): 1394–401, 1401.e1–4.

Tomiyama, A. Janet, Mary F. Dallman, Ph.D., and Elissa S. Epel. "Comfort Food Is Comforting to Those Most Stressed: Evidence of the Chronic

Stress Response Network in High Stress Women." *Psychoneuroendocrinology* 36 (2011): 1513–19.

Truelove, Sidney C. "Movements of the Large Intestine." *Physiological Reviews* 46 (1966): 457–512.

Trust for America's Health Foundation and Robert Wood Johnson Foundation. "Obesity Rates and Trends: Adult Obesity in the US." http: //state ofobesity.org/rates/ (accessed September 2015)

Ursell, Luke K., Henry J. Haiser, Will Van Treuren, Neha Garg, Lavanya Reddivari, Jairam Vanamala, Pieter C. Dorrestein, Peter J. Turnbaugh, and Rob Knight. "The Intestinal Metabolome: An Intersection Between Microbiota and Host." *Gastroenterology* 146 (2014): 1470–76.

Vals-Pedret, Cinta, Aleix Sala-Vila, DPharm, Mercè Serra-Mir, Dolores Corella, DPharm, Rafael de la Torre, Miguel Ángel Martínez-González, Elena H. Martínez-Lapiscina, et al. "Mediterranean Diet and Age-Related Cognitive Decline: A Randomized Clinical Trial." *Journal of the American Medical Association Internal Medicine* 175 (2015): 1094–1103.

Van Oudenhove, Lukas, Shane McKie, Daniel Lassman, Bilal Uddin, Peter Paine, Steven Coen, Lloyd Gregory, Jan Tack, and Qasim Aziz. "Fatty Acid–Induced Gut-Brain Signaling Attenuates Neural and Behavioral Effects of Sad Emotion in Humans." *Journal of Clinical Investigation* 121 (2011): 3094–99.

Volkow, Nora D., Gene-Jack Wangc, Dardo Tomasib, and Ruben D. Balera. "The Addictive Dimensionality of Obesity." *Biological Psychiatry* 73 (2013): 811–18.

Walsh, John H. "Gastrin (First of Two Parts)." *New England Journal of Medicine* 292 (1975): 1324–34.

———. "Peptides as Regulators of Gastric Acid Secretion." *Annual Review of Physiology* 50 (1998): 41–63.

Weltens, N., D. Zhao, and Lukas Van Oudenhove. "Where is the Comfort in Comfort Foods? Mechanisms Linking Fat Signaling, Reward, and Emotion." *Neurogastroenterology and Motility* 26 (2014): 303–15.

Wu, Gary D., Jun Chen, Christian Hoffmann, Kyle Bittinger, Ying-Yu Chen, Sue A. Keilbaugh, Meenakshi Bewtra, et al. "Linking Long-Term Dietary Patterns with Gut Microbial Enterotypes." *Science* 334 (2011): 105–8.

Wu, Gary D., Charlene Compher, Eric Z. Chen, Sarah A. Smith, Rachana D. Shah, Kyle Bittinger, Christel Chehoud, et al. "Comparative Metabolomics in Vegans and Omnivores Reveal Constraints on Diet-Dependent Gut Microbiota Metabolite Production." *Gut* 65 (2016): 63–72.

Yano, Jessica M., Kristie Yu, Gregory P. Donaldson, Gauri G. Shastri, Phoebe Ann, Liang Ma, Cathryn R. Nagler, Rustem F. Ismagilov, Sarkis K.

Mazmanian, and Elaine Y. Hsiao. "Indigenous Bacteria from the Gut Microbiota Regulate Host Serotonin Biosynthesis." *Cell* 161 (2015): 264–76.

Yatsunenko, Tanya, Federico E. Rey, Mark J. Manary, Indi Trehan, Maria Gloria Dominguez-Bello, Monica Contreras, Magda Magris, et al. "Human Gut Microbiome Viewed Across Age and Geography." *Nature* 486 (2012): 222–27.

Zeevi, David, Tal Korem, Niv Zmora, David Israeli, Daphna Rothschild, Adina Weinberger, Orly Ben-Yacov, et al. "Personalized Nutrition by Prediction of Glycemic Responses." *Cell* 163 (2015): 1079–94.

Zheng, P., B. Zeng, C. Zhou, M. Liu, Z. Fang, X. Xu, L. Zeng, J. Chen, S. Fan, X. Du, X. Zhang, D. Yang, Y. Yang, H. Meng, W. Li, N. D. Melgiri, J. Licinio, H. Wei, and P. Xie. "Gut Microbiome Remodeling Induces Depressive-Like Behaviors through a Pathway Mediated by the Host's Metabolism." *Molecular Psychiatry* 21 (2016):786–796.

INDEX

||||||||||||||||||||||

Page numbers of illustrations appear in italics.

ABOUT THE AUTHOR

||||||||||||||||||||||||||||||||||||||||||||||||||||||||||||||||||||||||

Emeran A. Mayer, MD, has studied brain body interactions for the last forty years, with a particular emphasis on brain-gut interactions. He is the executive director of the Oppenheimer Center for Stress and Resilience and the codirector of the Digestive Diseases Research Center at the University of California at Los Angeles. His research has been supported by the National Institutes of Health for the past twenty-five years, and he is considered a pioneer and world leader in the areas of brain-gut microbiome interactions and chronic visceral pain. He has appeared on National Public Radio (NPR), on PBS, and in the documentary *In Search of Balance*. His work has been written about in the *Atlantic*, *Scientific American*, the *New York Times*, the *Guardian*, among other publications. He lives in Los Angeles.